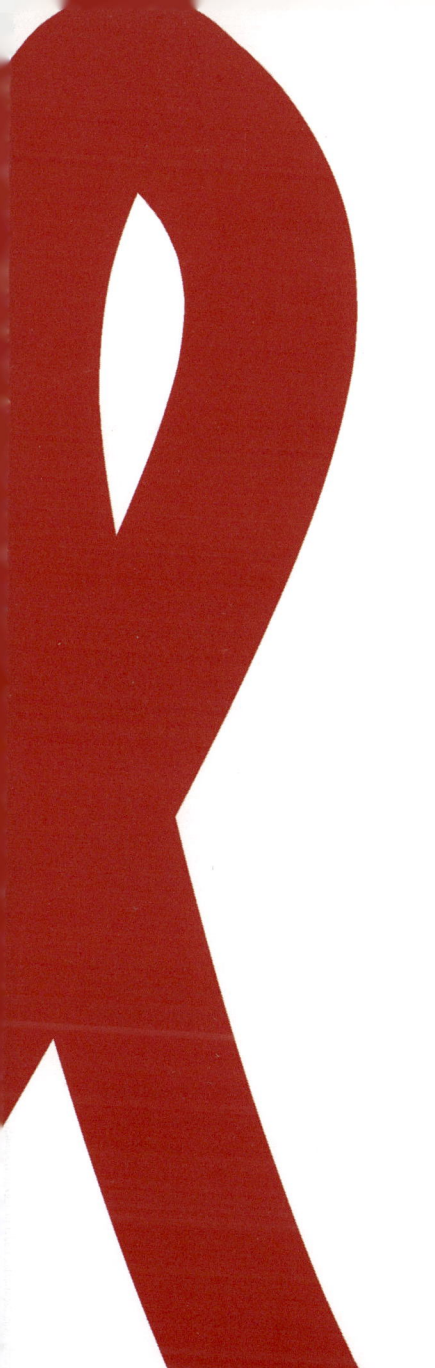

Corporate
Responses
to HIV/AIDS

Case Studies from India

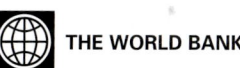
THE WORLD BANK

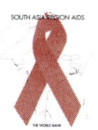
WORLD BANK INSTITUTE
Promoting knowledge and learning for a better world

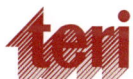

Manufactured in India
Second printing October 2007

This volume is a product of the staff of the International Bank for Reconstruction and Development/The World Bank. The findings, interpretations, and conclusions expressed in this paper do not necessarily reflect the views of the Executive Directors of The World Bank or the governments they represent.

The findings, interpretations, and conclusions expressed in this book are entirely those of the authors and should not be attributed in any manner to the World Bank, to its affiliated organizations, or to members of its Board of Executive Directors or the countries they represent. The World Bank does not guarantee the accuracy of the data included in this publication and accepts no responsibility for any consequence of their use. The boundaries, colors, denominations, and other information shown on any map in this volume do not imply on the part of the World Bank Group any judgment on the legal status of any territory or the endorsement or acceptance of such boundaries.

ISBN-10: 0-8213-7171-1
ISBN-13: 978-0-8213-7171-8
e-ISBN: 0-8213-7172-X
DOI: 10.1596/978-0-8213-7171-8

Library of Congress Cataloging-in-Publication Data has been applied for.

Design and layout: James E. Quigley, World Bank Institute

Photos courtesy of the World Bank, Reliance Industries Limited, Transport Corporation of India Limited, Delhi Metro Rail Corporation, DCM Shriram Consolidated Limited, and Hindustan Lever Limited.

Contents

Case Study: Hindustan Lever Limited............................75

References..87

Tables

Figures

Boxes

Pictures

Foreword

Businesses suffer from the effects of HIV and AIDS, but they can fight back. Corporations can take decisive early action to prevent HIV and reduce stigma—before the epidemic becomes generalized in the population and more difficult and costly to control. Businesses interact with most people in a country—directly, with employees, as well as more indirectly, with employees' families and with customers and community members. By playing a more active role, together with government and civil society, companies have an opportunity to exercise leadership in a way that helps millions and makes both business and moral sense.

At the micro level the impact of AIDS on enterprises—through their employers, managers, and workers—is well documented where the epidemic has hit hardest. In those areas AIDS increases the cost of doing business, and companies are recognizing that becoming involved in stemming the spread of the epidemic is good not only for corporate citizenship but also for corporate self-interest, even survival.

AIDS has a direct impact on companies' profitability. In the worst-case scenario the economic effects are observed in greater absenteeism and staff turnover, higher recruitment and training costs, and higher costs in medical care or insurance coverage, retirement funds or funeral fees. A less obvious but equally important cost is declining morale and productivity among employees. AIDS not only affects the health of workers; it also takes a toll on their savings, the resources of their families, and their productivity as they start spending more time taking care of the sick. In India this scenario can be prevented by businesses taking bold action now.

At the macro level HIV and AIDS hit hardest among those in their most productive years, ages 15–24. Evidence from other parts of the world suggests that India's booming and talented workforce is becoming increasingly vulnerable to the virus as people become more mobile, lifestyles change, and disposable incomes rise. This is important not only to the information technology and business service companies but to the country as a whole—because it is young adults who are the driving force behind India's impressive growth today and its potential growth and prosperity in the coming years.

The government of India has taken significant measures to curb the spread of HIV, at both national and state levels. But much remains to be done. Businesses can play an important part, particularly in HIV prevention but also in care and treatment of AIDS patients.

This collection of case studies aims to contribute to the growing evidence on private sector engagement in the fight against HIV and AIDS and the challenges businesses are overcoming in this fight. By capturing the experiences of the local private sector, it seeks to foster a more active response from the business community and to encourage new partnership approaches from government, civil society, and development organizations to leverage the goodwill and competencies of the private sector. In a country as large as India, more active engagement of the private sector is critical to achieve the scale of intervention needed to get ahead of HIV and AIDS. We hope the lessons of these case studies will be of interest not only to private and public partners in India but also to partners in other countries in South Asia and beyond.

Praful Patel
Vice President
World Bank South Asia Region

Simon Bell
Sector Manager
South Asia Finance and Private Sector

Acknowledgments

This report was prepared by the World Bank's South Asia Finance and Private Sector (SASFP) unit and the South Asia Regional AIDS (SAR AIDS) team, in collaboration with the Business, Competitiveness, and Development team of the World Bank Institute (WBI) and The Energy and Resources Institute (TERI). The report team was led by Samuel Munzele Maimbo, Shanthi Divakaran, and Mehmet Can Atacik in collaboration with Jenny Gold. Overall guidance was provided by Mariam Claeson, Simon Bell and Djordjija Petkoski. TERI members included Swetha Dasari and Satyajeet Subramanian, under the guidance of Annapurna Vancheswaran. At various stages the team received valuable inputs from Hnin Hnin Pyne, Suneeta Singh, and Sabine Durier. The draft report benefited greatly from the review and comments received from Sujatha Rao (National AIDS Control Organization), and Gina Dallabetta (Bill & Melinda Gates Foundation). The report was edited by Alison Strong and designed by James Quigley. Maria Marjorie Espiritu provided administrative support.

Acronyms and Abbreviations

AIDS	Acquired immunodeficiency syndrome
DMRC	Delhi Metro Rail Corporation
DOTS	Directly Observed Treatment, Short-course
DSCL	DCM Shriram Consolidated Limited
FHI	Family Health International
GSNP+	Gujarat State Network of People Living with HIV
HIV	Human immunodeficiency virus
HLL	Hindustan Lever Limited
ILO	International Labour Organization
JBIC	Japan Bank for International Cooperation
LVS	Lok Vikas Sanstha
NACO	National AIDS Control Organization
NACP	National AIDS Control Program
NGO	Nongovernmental organization
NH	National highway
PATH	Program for Appropriate Technology in Health
PSI	Population Services International

RIL	Reliance Industries Limited
Rs	Rupees
STD	Sexually transmitted disease
STI	Sexually transmitted infection
TB	Tuberculosis
TCI	Transport Corporation of India
UNAIDS	Joint United Nations Programme on HIV/AIDS
WHO	World Health Organization

Executive Summary

Businesses have an enormous stake in the fight against HIV and AIDS, an epidemic that affects their workforce and, if left unchecked, can rob them of their workers and their markets. They stand to gain from supporting interventions aimed at preventing HIV both at the workplace and in local communities—and from taking early decisive action while there is still opportunity to prevent a generalized epidemic. Moreover, businesses bring critical advantages to these efforts, including management skills, resources, and influence over the general workforce.

Lessons from HIV and AIDS interventions by Indian businesses

In India both private and public sector companies are pursuing notable programs of HIV and AIDS awareness and prevention for employees and for local communities. All these programs have faced challenges. The ways they have addressed those challenges offer lessons that may be useful to other interventions by private and public sector businesses, both current and future:

1

- *Leveraging partnerships.* Partnerships with local NGOs, State AIDS Control Societies, and other agencies have proved critical to the success of several programs. One program, for example, developed its approach to HIV prevention through discussions with the State AIDS Control Society and broadened its outreach by partnering with an active network of people living with HIV. Programs operating clinics along national highways for long-distance truckers depend on partnerships with local NGOs across the country. Others rely on construction contractors to ensure that migrant workers are exposed to HIV and AIDS awareness programs.

- *Communicating messages effectively.* Companies have used several approaches to communicate HIV and AIDS messages to their workforce and local communities. One company in this collection of case studies customizes information, education, and communication material in imaginative ways to capture the attention of its target audience—producing cassettes that intersperse HIV and AIDS messages with popular Hindi film songs and having talented employees convey messages through songs and poems at company events. Most such communication efforts, however, need better monitoring and evaluation to assess their effectiveness in changing attitudes and practices.

- *Keeping up with highly mobile target groups.* Many target groups, such as sex workers and their clients, are highly mobile. To support and track one such group, long-distance truckers, one program operating clinics along highways issues each participating trucker a "passport" recording the trucker's medical history. Truckers present their passport on each visit to any of the clinics, allowing them easy access to services and giving medical staff easy access to their medical history.

- *Coping with poor public health infrastructure.* Lack of government health facilities has created challenges in several cases. One program has found that because government medical and testing facilities are closed on weekends, laborers often turn to fake doctors. Mobile health clinics could help overcome this challenge by providing laborers easier access to medical services on weekdays.
- *Countering social stigma.* Predictably, most programs have encountered resistance to HIV and AIDS messages because of the stigma attached to the epidemic and to topics related to sex. Programs have had to use repeated awareness programs to encourage employees to pick up free condoms. And among those that have set up medical centers to treat AIDS patients, one had to address concerns among villagers that a center's proximity to their homes could expose them to contagious diseases.
- *Overcoming message fatigue and negative branding.* Programs targeted to truckers found that messages became ineffective with too much repetition. Moreover, repeated interventions targeted to truckers saddled them with negative branding because of the stigma associated with HIV and AIDS. To counter these effects, one program, for example, has experimented with theater performances featuring truckers as protagonists while communicating HIV and AIDS messages.

The approaches used by five Indian companies

This report features five case studies illustrating approaches that private and public sector companies have used in HIV and AIDS interventions. Other companies in India have pursued similar activities. Through the "IFC Against AIDS" program, for example, the International Finance

Corporation, a member of the World Bank Group, works with four Indian companies implementing HIV and AIDS interventions: Ambuja Cement, Apollo Tyres, Ballarpur Industries Limited (BILT), and Usha Martin.[1] The details and lessons of these interventions and those of the five case studies in this report may be helpful to other companies designing or implementing HIV and AIDS interventions for their workforce and communities.

The interventions of the five companies highlighted in the report have ranged from advocacy and generation of awareness to prevention and treatment (table 1):

- *Reliance Industries Limited*, India's largest private company, set up a well-equipped medical center near its industrial site in Hazira, Gujarat, where it provides both tuberculosis and AIDS treatment. Since inception of the program in 2004, company physicians and local NGOs have together reached nearly 300,000 people through awareness initiatives, testing and counseling services, and antiretroviral therapy.
- *Transport Corporation of India (TCI)*, recognizing the importance of truckers to its business and the vulnerability of the trucking community to HIV and AIDS, established a network of clinics along national highways. Operated by local NGOs, these clinics serve long-distance truck drivers and their assistants, providing treatment for sexually transmitted infections and counseling services aimed at preventing HIV.
- *Delhi Metro Rail Corporation (DMRC)*, a public sector company, is constructing the metro rail system in Delhi. This enormous construction project draws migrant workers, a population typically at high risk for HIV infection, from across India. DMRC initiated an

---

1. International Finance Corporation, "IFC Against AIDS: Projects," http://www.ifc.org/ifcext/aids.nsf/Content/Projects.

HIV and AIDS program for contractors and workers that included advocacy, peer education, and promotion of condom use. This nine-month program reached more than 3,000 workers. The company has ensured that the efforts will be extended: its agreements with contractors now require that they carry out HIV prevention activities for employees working on DMRC projects.

- *DCM Shriram Consolidated Limited (DSCL)*, a company with interests mainly in chemicals and agribusiness, initiated an HIV and AIDS program at its plant in Kota, Rajasthan, aimed at providing a safe and healthy work environment. The program draws on the local culture, adapting information, education, and communication material to local sensibilities and using cultural performances to convey HIV and AIDS messages. This strategy has helped broaden the appeal of its messages and gain acceptance for the program among the local population.

- *Hindustan Lever Limited (HLL)*, a fast-moving consumer goods company with more than a hundred manufacturing plants across India, has initiated workplace programs aimed at protecting the health of its skilled young workforce. With technical assistance from the International Labour Organization, the company's factories have built HIV and AIDS awareness programs into their health and safety training. HLL has also used its expertise in distribution and management to spread HIV and AIDS awareness through initiatives with rural entrepreneurs. And in the future it plans to use its extensive marketing network in rural areas to promote use of condoms.

Table 1. Summary of the case studies

Company	Industry	Location of intervention	Intervention areas	Beneficiaries	Partners
Reliance Industries Limited	Petrochemicals, textiles, others	Hazira, Gujarat	Awareness and prevention, HIV testing, treatment for AIDS, advocacy	Contract workers, migrant workers, truckers, employees, local community, local enterprises	Confederation Indian Indust Gujarat State AIDS Control Society, Guja State Networ of People Livi with HIV, Lok Samarpan, Lo Vikas Sansth Reliance Life Sciences
Transport Corporation of India	Cargo transport	Andhra Pradesh, Delhi, Jharkhand, Karnataka, Madhya Pradesh, Maharashtra, Orissa, Rajasthan, Uttar Pradesh	Awareness and prevention, treatment for sexually transmitted infections, advocacy	Long-distance truckers, local community	Avahan, CARI Family Health International, Population Se vices International, Progra for Appropriat Technology in Health (PATH)
Delhi Metro Rail Corporation	Public transport	Delhi	Awareness and prevention, advocacy	Migrant workers employed by contractors	International Labour Organ zation, Japan Bank for Inter tional Cooper tion, Modicar Foundation
DCM Shriram Consolidated Limited	Agribusiness, chemicals, plastics, others	Kota, Rajasthan	Awareness and prevention, treatment for AIDS, advocacy	Employees, contract workers, truckers, local community	Confederation Indian Indust The Energy an Resources In tute, Rajastha State AIDS Co trol Society
Hindustan Lever Limited	Fast-moving consumer goods	Southern, eastern, western, and northern corporate regions[a]	Awareness and prevention, HIV testing, advocacy	Employees, contract workers, truckers, local and rural communities	Confederation Indian Indust International Labour Organ zation, Nation AIDS Control ganization, lo NGOs, hospit

a. Hindustan Lever Limited's southern region encompasses Andhra Pradesh, Karnataka, Kerala, and Tamil Nadu (prog activities reported from Karnataka and Tamil Nadu); its eastern region, seven northeastern states along with Ass Jharkhand, Orissa, and West Bengal (program activities reported from Assam); and its northern region, Delhi, Hima Pradesh, Jammu and Kashmir, Punjab, Rajasthan, Uttaranchal, and Uttar Pradesh.

Key recommendations

Experience in combating HIV and AIDS in India points to several key recommendations for private and public sector programs:

- *Take early decisive action.* Companies that carry out HIV and AIDS interventions do so to safeguard the health of their employees and because these efforts accord with their values and mission. Such efforts can meet resistance—at the corporate level, at the workplace, and in the local community—especially where action is taken early to stem an epidemic before it has become generalized, when the perceived risk may be low. But taking early decisive action on prevention before the epidemic gets out of control pays off for companies: it reduces the future burden of death and disability and averts the high cost of treating and caring for large numbers of people living with AIDS.
- *Document cost and effectiveness.* There is much to learn from actions taken by businesses to prevent HIV and treat and care for AIDS patients. It is important to learn by doing. But beyond this, formal, independent evaluation is needed to assess the effectiveness of these interventions. Better monitoring and evaluation will help in planning and implementing programs, in identifying gaps, and, importantly, in sustaining, scaling up, and expanding initiatives.
- *Ensure sustained commitment and financing.* A challenge for both the private and the public sector is to sustain the financing for prevention, treatment, and care. Continued financing is especially essential for treatment programs, which, once initiated, must not be interrupted. Developing strategies for sustaining programs—whether run by businesses or by government—will become increasingly important, providing a strong impetus for greater private-public partnership and sharing of knowledge.

Introduction

Indian businesses have become an important stakeholder in the fight against HIV and AIDS. According to the National AIDS Control Organization, 5.2 million adults ages 15–49 in India are HIV-positive, representing one-eighth of global HIV cases (Chandrasekaran and others 2006). A large share of this HIV-positive population are employees of Indian industry.

The case for business involvement

India has maintained an average annual growth rate of more than 7 percent in the decade since 1994,[2] and by January 2006 had built up its foreign exchange reserves to more than US$139 billion (India, Ministry of Finance 2006). The country also is becoming a leading destination for foreign investment. But while Indian industry has been growing at an impressive pace, it faces potentially large risks from increasing social challenges.

---

2. U.S. Central Intelligence Agency, "India: Economy Overview," in The World Factbook, https://www.cia.gov/cia/publications/factbook/geos/in.html (last accessed November 15, 2006).

Particularly alarming are the potential repercussions of the HIV and AIDS epidemic. India does not have the high prevalence of HIV infection that African countries do, but it has the second largest number of people living with HIV and AIDS after South Africa. Moreover, India's population, already more than one billion, is expected to surpass China's by 2010. In this scenario even a small increase in the prevalence rate could mean a staggering number of infections.

Already HIV has spread across the nation, reaching both urban and rural pockets. While India faces mainly concentrated epidemics, among high-risk groups, several states face generalized epidemics (Moses and others 2006). The groups most at risk are sex workers and their clients, many of whom are migrant workers, truckers, and others who spend long periods away from home; injecting drug users and their sexual partners; and men having sex with men. For India the challenge of fighting the epidemic is made even more daunting by illiteracy, mass poverty, and socioeconomic disparities between men and women, all of which contribute to HIV and AIDS.

AIDS kills primarily young and middle-aged adults during their peak productive years. By reducing the labor supply and disposable incomes, a generalized epidemic can have broad macroeconomic effects, dampening markets, savings rates, investment, and consumer spending. Assessing the economic impact of AIDS is difficult. But studies suggest that some of the hardest-hit countries with generalized epidemics may forfeit 2 percent or more of annual GDP growth (World Bank 2006).

As India becomes a global economic power, it is important that Indian businesses continue to bear in mind their corporate social responsibility, pursuing business practices and policies that are in the best interest of the community at large. Businesses have much to gain from early decisive action to prevent HIV and reduce the cost and social impact of AIDS.

The heterogeneous nature of the epidemic in India suggests that there is no one strategy for Indian businesses in the fight against HIV and AIDS. Businesses that employ groups most at risk, such as truckers, may need to implement targeted interventions. But all businesses can contribute to curbing the epidemic through a set of activities that include the following:

- Generating awareness about HIV and AIDS.
- Reducing stigma (for example, destigmatizing HIV testing by promoting an HIV testing day or having a high-profile person in the company be publicly tested).
- Pursuing high-level advocacy efforts (such as by having corporate leaders speak publicly about HIV and AIDS).
- Creating an HIV policy for the workplace.
- Providing referrals for counseling and testing.

What industry gains from setting up HIV and AIDS programs

The HIV epidemic can have a direct impact on businesses through its effect on their workforce. Yet in India only a small share of the private sector—around 70 companies—are engaged in fighting HIV and AIDS.[3] Farsighted companies have incorporated the fight against HIV and AIDS into their corporate strategy because they are convinced that there is a business case for doing so:

- *Control of the cost of HIV and AIDS.* While India has a relatively low national prevalence of HIV, prevalence rates vary (from high to low) between and within states, and the total number of HIV-positive people is high. HIV and AIDS can impose large costs on

---

3. Based on discussion with the HIV and AIDS team of the International Labour Organization, Delhi, on November 14, 2005.

businesses through higher medical and health insurance spending and the need to recruit and train new staff to replace those who are lost. Where prevalence rates are high, the epidemic also leads to higher costs, and to lower revenues, as a result of greater absenteeism and staff turnover, lower productivity, declining morale, and a shrinking consumer base. Where the epidemic continues to grow, companies may face a shortage of healthy labor in the long run, leading to a migration of workers between cities and states to fill labor needs. Companies would have to bear the long-term cost of this migration, including the cost of relocating staff and providing housing and other benefits.

- *Conflict reduction in the workplace.* Within companies a lack of awareness and understanding of HIV and AIDS can lead to conflict in the workplace and thus disruptions for management. HIV and AIDS awareness programs can help reduce these conflicts that arise because of lack of information and communication.

- *Strong markets.* Businesses survive and succeed in settings where people have the capacity to purchase. In regions heavily affected by HIV and AIDS the general pattern of expenditure is skewed toward health care and medication. It is thus in the interest of businesses to stem the spread of the epidemic so as to retain and build markets for their products and services.

- *General goodwill and better relations with stakeholders.* The danger of HIV and AIDS has raised concern throughout society. Thus companies that launch HIV prevention programs gain from the publicity benefits of engaging in corporate social responsibility. Establishing an HIV and AIDS program also improves relations with labor and with other key stakeholders, such as investors, the government, and civil society.

What advantages businesses bring to the fight

Businesses, particularly private sector ones, have been an effective partner in addressing HIV and AIDS in South Asia. Companies have many comparative advantages that they can mobilize in the fight against AIDS:

- *Coverage and influence.* A large share of the HIV-affected population work for businesses, giving these businesses significant influence over the general workforce. Businesses can harness this influence to spread HIV and AIDS education and awareness among employees and their families. Their organizational structure also provides mechanisms for reaching out to a larger group of people. Firms have influence over supply chain networks and other players with links to the general workforce. Thus companies that want to extend their efforts beyond their own workplace can develop ways to encourage their suppliers and distributors to help prevent the spread of HIV. The influence of businesses in mainstreaming HIV and AIDS initiatives is also important in reducing stigma.
- *Lobbying power.* Businesses have the power to form strong lobby groups that can influence government policy. Collectively, Indian companies could work through business associations and councils to promote HIV prevention programs at the workplace in all sectors. They could also raise and donate funds for strengthening communications infrastructure and connectivity to provide easy access to useful information on HIV and AIDS.
- *Special expertise.* Private companies generally have the managerial skills to run a program more effectively than the public sector. They offer a range of capabilities—logistics expertise, technical know-how, financial and accounting skills, and communications, media, marketing, and training skills. All these can be brought to bear in changing opinions, attitudes, and behaviors on a large

scale so as to reduce the stigma associated with HIV and AIDS and stem the spread of the epidemic.

- *Financial resources.* Private firms typically have the financial resources and infrastructure to carry out HIV and AIDS interventions such as awareness programs. They can also find innovative ways to finance and sustain programs.
- *Results orientation.* The private sector's typically higher efficiency (compared with the public sector's) could help in achieving more efficient and effective HIV and AIDS interventions, if well monitored and evaluated.

How the Indian government supports companies involved in HIV and AIDS interventions

India has both national and state organizational structures for combating HIV and AIDS. At the national level the government has established the multisector National Council on AIDS, chaired by the prime minister. At the state level each State AIDS Council is chaired by the state's chief minister and the vice chair of its Ministry of Health.

In addition, the Indian government leads a broad-based national program on HIV and AIDS through the National AIDS Control Organization, a semiautonomous agency set up in the Ministry of Health in 1992.[4] This agency, along with the local State AIDS Control Societies, has a role in steering the fight against HIV. It has a dedicated senior core staff

4. National AIDS Control Organization, "About NACO," http://nacoonline.org/abt_faq. htm (last accessed November 15, 2006).

whose work includes mainstreaming HIV and AIDS prevention, treatment, and care; developing capacity; and providing hands-on support across sectors. The national program includes:

- Targeted interventions for HIV and AIDS prevention and awareness.
- Control of sexually transmitted infections (STIs).
- Information, education, and communication.
- Treatment, care, and support for AIDS patients.
- Training (such as for medical and paramedical staff of blood banks and for NGOs or companies implementing HIV and AIDS programs).
- Sentinel surveillance (monitoring of HIV infection trends in specific high- and low-risk groups).[5]
- Program management.
- Advocacy and social mobilization.
- Strategies and interventions for blood safety and training.

The National AIDS Control Organization and local State AIDS Control Societies have partnered with several Indian industry coalitions and companies in carrying out HIV and AIDS interventions.

---

5. In India sentinel surveillance of high-risk groups includes people attending drug addiction treatment centers, clinics for sexually transmitted infections, and clinics for men having sex with men. Low-risk segments include mothers attending prenatal clinics, a category taken as a proxy for the general population (National AIDS Control Organization, "Facts and Figures: An Overview of the Spread and Prevalence of HIV/AIDS in India," http://www.nacoonline.org/facts_overview.htm, last accessed November 15, 2006).

The case studies

Among the Indian companies already engaged in the fight against HIV and AIDS, what shape do their efforts take and what are the lessons of their experience? To find out, case studies were conducted to highlight the work of companies promoting HIV and AIDS awareness and providing HIV- and AIDS-related services at the workplace and in local communities.

To identify the case studies, a shortlist was prepared of companies that had HIV and AIDS programs with clear objectives and dedicated resources, including staff and infrastructure. From this shortlist five companies were selected that reflect a variety of sectors, partnership models, target groups, and intervention mechanisms:

- Reliance Industries Limited.
- Transport Corporation of India.
- Delhi Metro Rail Corporation.
- DCM Shriram Consolidated Limited.
- Hindustan Lever Limited.

All the companies except Delhi Metro Rail Corporation are in the private sector.

The case studies were researched using a mix of methods: standard questionnaires administered to companies; meetings with senior management, human resource personnel, and corporate social responsibility teams at factory locations or the corporate office; telephone interviews; review of internal documents; and written correspondence.

The case studies illustrate the importance of integrating multiple stakeholders in the fight against HIV and AIDS. They also highlight the growing investment of businesses in that fight—an investment that recognizes their vulnerability to the economic and social impact of the epidemic. And they show what businesses can achieve by tackling HIV and AIDS through the workforce.

Each of the five businesses contributes its unique perspective, expertise, and skills to helping to curb the HIV and AIDS epidemic in the microcosm in which it operates. By showcasing their achievements and illuminating the lessons of their experience, these case studies seek to convince other businesses that taking part in the fight against HIV and AIDS is both within their reach and in their interest.

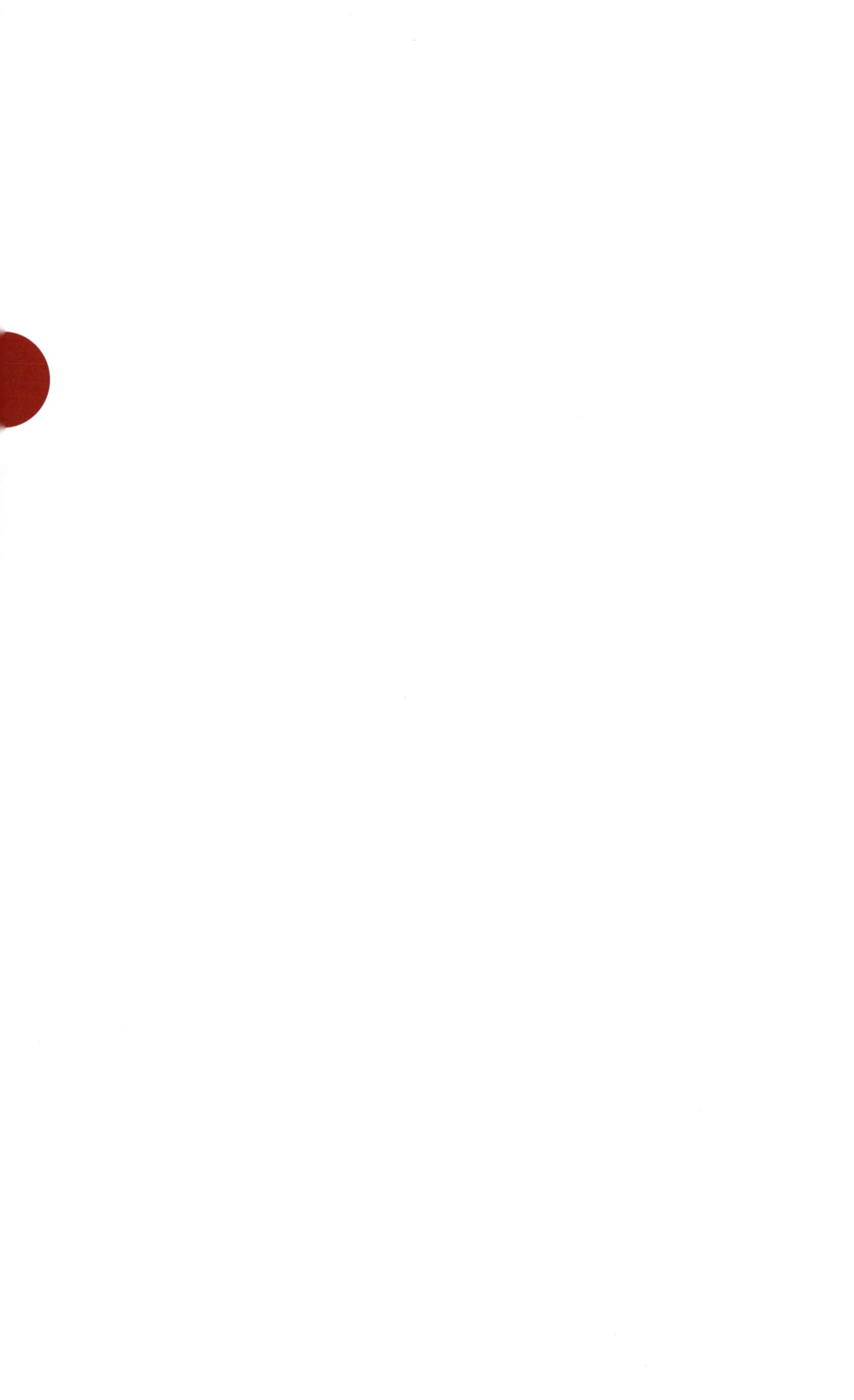

Case Study:
Reliance Industries Limited

Overview

Reliance Industries Limited is India's largest private enterprise, with businesses straddling several sectors and a workforce of 25,000 employees.[6] Its large workforce and extensive operations give it a big stake in the fight against HIV and AIDS.

The company's HIV and AIDS program is unusual among those initiated by private companies in India in that it not only promotes awareness of HIV and AIDS but also provides treatment. Another unique feature of the program is its broad coverage: it provides antiretroviral therapy to anyone in the community who is HIV-positive, whether or not that person is an employee of the company.

The program began by establishing a well-equipped health center at Hazira, in Gujarat, to provide tuberculosis treatment based on the strategy recommended by the World Health Organization (WHO), known as DOTS (Directly Observed Treatment, Short-course). The center, which

---

6. The information in the Reliance case study is based on personal interviews with Reliance officials responsible for the company's HIV and AIDS program, site visits, and internal documents shared by the company. The information is current as of September 2006.

also offered information on HIV prevention, later expanded to treatment and other services for AIDS patients. It also provides counseling, education, and training and disseminates information on nutrition.

Reliance has worked closely with partners to help extend the program's reach. In villages near Hazira local NGOs disseminate information and refer HIV-positive people to the center. While education programs and the center itself initially encountered resistance because of the social stigma associated with HIV and AIDS, repeated awareness activities have helped gain acceptance.

The program has already reached nearly 300,000 people—truckers (drivers and crew members), contract and migrant workers, employees of local enterprises, and members of the local community. Reliance is now initiating a process of replicating the program at other company sites.

Business background

Reliance is a big presence in the Indian economy, with annual sales of US$20 billion, a net worth of US$11 billion, and total assets of US$21 billion. Its activities include oil and gas exploration and production, petroleum refining and marketing, petrochemicals (polyester, fiber intermediates, plastics, and chemicals), and textiles. Its exports reach nearly 100 countries across the globe, totaling US$7 billion annually.

The company operates manufacturing facilities at several sites in Gujarat. The Naroda facility, near Ahmedabad, houses a textile plant. The Pa-

> As a global business leader, we are equally concerned about the society we live in and our environment. We have constantly pursued businesses that will trigger high growth and promote sustainable development, and this has been and must continue to be one of our guiding philosophies.
>
> —Mukesh D. Ambani, Chairman
> Reliance Industries

talganga complex, near Mumbai, has polyester, fiber intermediate, and linear alkyl benzene manufacturing plants. The Hazira complex, near Surat, has a naphtha cracker feeding downstream fiber intermediate, plastics, and polyester plants. And the Jamnagar complex has a petroleum refinery and associated petrochemical plants that produce plastics and fiber intermediates.

Why do something about HIV and AIDS?

As an industrial site, Hazira has a large migrant workforce employed in several local industries. The presence of these industries has also contributed to a large, floating population of truckers in Hazira. Concerned about the risk of infectious diseases in such a population, the local government sought corporate support to set up HIV and tuberculosis programs at the workplace and in medical camps in local villages and on local highways.

In 2004 the district tuberculosis program approached Reliance about collaborating in efforts to address tuberculosis in Hazira. Around the same time, at the World Economic Forum, Reliance committed to working toward combating HIV and AIDS in India. Together, these two events gave management the impetus to initiate a full-time HIV and tuberculosis program at the company's Hazira location.

The company's management began by discussing possible intervention strategies with Lok Vikas Sanstha (LVS), a local NGO specializing in public health. In 2004 LVS had conducted a baseline survey on the prevalence of sexually transmitted infections in Hazira and found that among the local population of migrant workers and truckers the prevalence rate was close to 12 percent (LVS 2004).

The discussions with LVS led Reliance to set up a DOTS tuberculosis and HIV center at Mora village on May 15, 2004, to provide medical services (both general and tuberculosis related) and information on HIV prevention for local villagers, truckers who halt for long hours, and the neighboring communities of migrant and contract workers. The center is housed in a community hall provided by Mora's *gram panchayat*.[7] Involving the panchayat helped create a sense of ownership among the local villagers.

The program

The Reliance HIV and AIDS program has two components: awareness and education, and treatment and support.

Awareness and education

Before launching its awareness program, Reliance held a series of discussions with the Gujarat State AIDS Control Society aimed at better understanding the nature of HIV prevalence in Hazira. These discussions made it clear that generating awareness among high-risk groups was a priority in stemming the spread of the epidemic. Reliance thus ensured that its awareness program extended beyond its employees and local villagers to high-risk groups in local industries.

Reliance employees

Reliance initiated the awareness program in-house, as part of its health, safety, and environment training for contract workers, supervisors, and

---

7. Every Indian village elects a panchayat, a five-person team that presides over the village's development affairs.

security staff. Conducted once a week by the company's on-site physician and LVS trainers, this training program has reached more than 5,000 workers. Besides basic information about preventing the transmission of HIV, sessions include discussions among workers to help clarify misperceptions about HIV and AIDS.

Initially those conducting the sessions faced challenges due to the strong stigma associated with HIV and AIDS. But Reliance has found that regular sessions and efforts to generate mass awareness among workers have substantially reduced fears relating to the epidemic.

Local community

Reliance has developed a multipronged approach to HIV and AIDS awareness and education in the local community. In nearby villages it conducts mass awareness programs through health camps. Sessions held at these camps discuss other health issues along with HIV, to diffuse the focus and

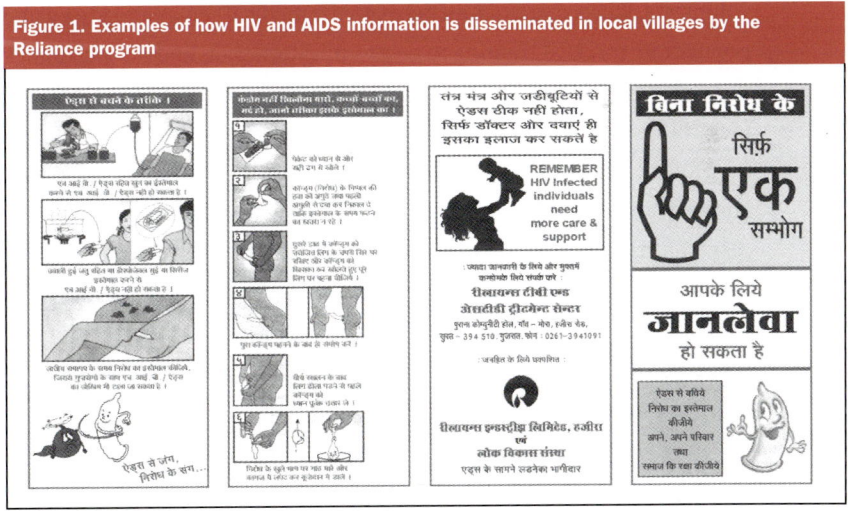

Figure 1. Examples of how HIV and AIDS information is disseminated in local villages by the Reliance program

thus lessen the discomfort of addressing HIV-related topics. A community mobilization team, with representatives from both Reliance and LVS, frequently visits neighboring villages (Damki, Suvali, Batlai, Junagaon, Vasva, and Rajgiri) to disseminate information (figure 2). Diagnostic and referral services are also provided in the health camps. Reliance bears the cost of both the health camps and any subsequent treatment.

As part of the effort to generate mass awareness, Reliance has also posted several educational banners in Surat and used street plays, poster exhibits, and video shows. Thanks to outreach efforts such as these, 25 HIV-positive sex workers from nearby villages are being monitored and treated by the medical center.

Reliance has also worked to generate awareness among truckers visiting its truck parking area, which draws nearly 1,000 trucks a day. Staff share information, distribute brochures printed in Hindi, Gujarati, and English, and hand out packs of condoms.

To strengthen its efforts in the community, Reliance has provided training to a group of young people who expressed interest in sharing information about HIV and AIDS with their neighbors and peers. These volunteers, who serve as a link between the medical center and the village population, received training in communication skills and on such topics as modes of HIV transmission, safe behavior, condom promotion, and identification of sexually transmitted infections.

Reliance has also provided training to local medical personnel aimed at increasing their awareness of and responsiveness to the concerns of HIV-positive people. The program has targeted doctors from urban health centers, the Employee State Insurance Scheme hospital, primary health centers of Surat district, and other private practitioners. Some 80 doctors and more than 100 paramedical staff have attended training programs.

Local enterprises

Having established awareness programs both at the company and in the local community, Reliance extended its efforts to high-risk groups in the local diamond and textile industries. These industries hire contract and migrant workers who live away from their families and in localities where prostitution is common, making them more susceptible to HIV infection.

In collaboration with the Confederation of Indian Industry, an association that represents industry on business and sustainable development issues, a team of Reliance and LVS staff visited a different enterprise each week to conduct HIV awareness sessions. A typical program would begin with a management meeting, followed by sensitization sessions with the workforce. It would conclude with the management signing an HIV and AIDS policy based on the International Labour Organization (ILO) workplace policy. In 2004–05 these sessions provided training to more than 8,000 workers in 67 textile and 24 diamond enterprises.

Treatment and support

Through its outreach activities Reliance discovered that Hazira and the nearby areas lacked adequate medical care and services for HIV-positive people. It therefore converted the DOTS tuberculosis and HIV center in Mora into an HIV testing, counseling, and treatment center offering a wide range of services. And it sent its physicians for special training on clinical intervention and softer skills needed to deal with HIV-positive patients.

The center provides a number of medical tests free for HIV-positive patients and at a heavily subsidized cost for others, including pregnancy tests, blood screening for syphilis (Venereal Disease Research Laboratory test), urine microscopy, and biochemical examinations such as liver function tests, blood sugar, and lipid profile. Patients seeking treatment for sexually transmitted infections receive counseling on such topics as modes of HIV transmission, the relationship between HIV and sexually transmitted infections, and the use of condoms. The center also provides antiretroviral therapy. And it offers emergency care including intravenous drugs and fluids and ambulance services.

Also among the services offered at the center are counseling, yoga training, pranayama coaching (breathing exercises to boost physical and mental spirits), and nutritional support. Malnutrition patients weighing less than 40 kilograms receive food and nutrition supplements.

Partnerships

Reliance management played a key leadership role in shaping the program and extending its outreach beyond company employees to the neighboring community. But partners have also been critical in implementing the program (figure 2):

- *Lok Vikas Sanstha*, through its team of 100 peer educators, has been responsible for organizing awareness campaigns in local areas and for the migrant workforce of Reliance on identification and treatment of sexually transmitted infections.
- *Gujarat State Network of People Living with HIV (GSNP+)*, an extremely active network of 1,600 members, has helped strengthen outreach by referring potential HIV-positive cases to the center. GSNP+ has provided counseling to HIV-positive people with no funds from Reliance. It encourages members of the network to take their medications regularly and coordinates with Reliance in providing medication and transport to the center. GSNP+ has also

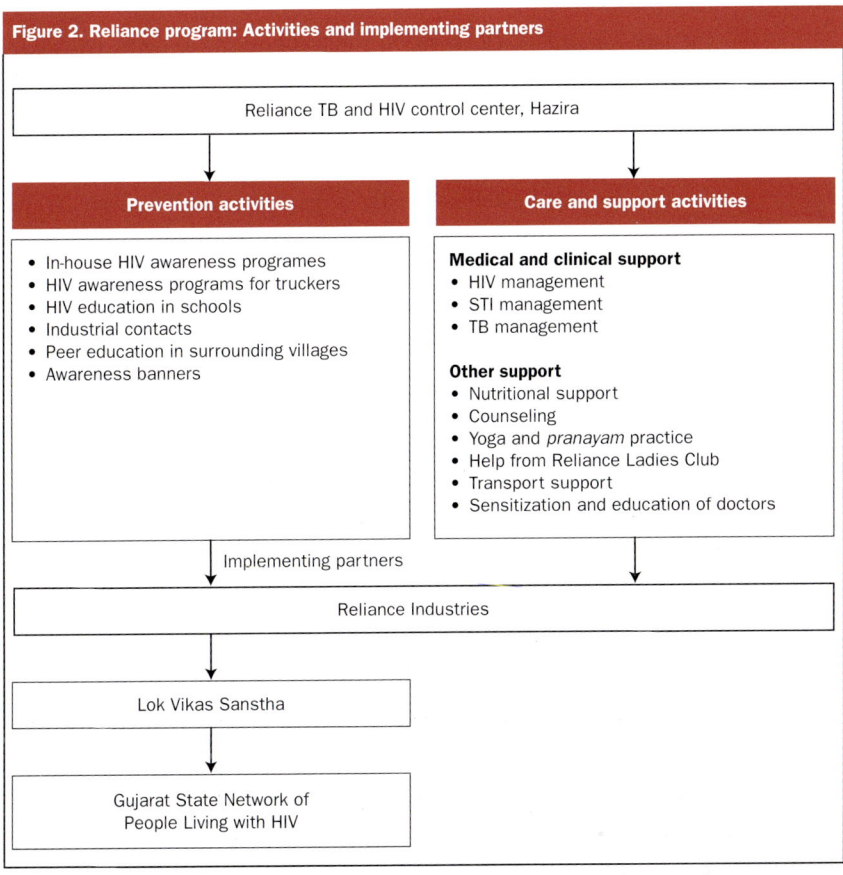

Figure 2. Reliance program: Activities and implementing partners

Reliance TB and HIV control center, Hazira

Prevention activities

- In-house HIV awareness programes
- HIV awareness programs for truckers
- HIV education in schools
- Industrial contacts
- Peer education in surrounding villages
- Awareness banners

Care and support activities

Medical and clinical support
- HIV management
- STI management
- TB management

Other support
- Nutritional support
- Counseling
- Yoga and *pranayam* practice
- Help from Reliance Ladies Club
- Transport support
- Sensitization and education of doctors

Implementing partners

Reliance Industries

Lok Vikas Sanstha

Gujarat State Network of People Living with HIV

worked with Reliance to sensitize local government authorities, which has led to the establishment of an AIDS information desk at the government hospital in Surat.

- *Reliance Life Sciences*, a research-oriented subsidiary in Mumbai focusing on medical, plant, and industrial biotechnology, has provided viral load testing (which determines the stage of HIV infections) at a subsidized cost.

- *Lok Samarpan*, a local blood bank, conducts CD4 tests (which report on the strength of the body's immune system and thus help assess the stage of the HIV infection and predict the risk of complications) at a subsidized rate of Rs 650 (US$14.50) per test. Further subsidy by Reliance reduces the cost to Rs 300 (US$6.50) per test. All costs are waived for widows and orphans.

Funding

In 2005–06 program costs amounted to Rs 100 lakhs (US$222,000). Reliance contributed Rs 75 lakhs (US$167,000), while the government covered the rest through the Gujarat State AIDS Control Society.

Outreach

The Reliance center has provided counseling to around 13,950 patients. Of these, 330 are patients receiving active antiretroviral therapy,[8] and 166 are tuberculosis patients receiving DOTS. In addition, 1,450 patients have been treated for sexually transmitted infections. A separate group of 626 HIV-positive patients are receiving regular monitoring and follow-up. The program has enabled nearly 250 HIV-positive people to return to regular work after beginning antiretroviral therapy.

Beyond the center, a mobile medical van pays weekly visits to nearby villages to offer free consultation and basic medication for general ailments. Between January 2005 and March 2006 this initiative benefited more than 140,000 villagers and 60,000 migrant workers.

---

8. The cost of providing antiretroviral therapy for one patient is Rs 1,500 (US$33) a month.

Lessons learned

The program has identified success factors, challenges, and lessons based on its experience.

Key success factors

- *Outreach.* In collaboration with program partners, the Reliance center has been able to provide quality services not only to company employees but also to a wide range of people in the community and at local enterprises. Indeed, patients from across southern Gujarat visit the center, some from as far as Amreli and Junagarh. The company attributes the success of its outreach efforts to the quality of services provided by the center and the referral network set up by partners.
- *NGO partnerships.* Top managers at Reliance have contributed greatly to the program's effectiveness through their involvement and commitment. But NGO partners have played a crucial role in enabling the program to expand and reach out to villagers, industrial workers, truckers, and the HIV-positive population.

Key challenges

- *Poor public health services.* The government's public health system often lacks the basic medical services and expertise required to administer quality care to AIDS patients. While this may not directly hinder operation of the center, an effective government system would help both support the services offered by the Reliance center and extend coverage to more patients.

- *Retention of village outreach workers.* Retaining village outreach workers has been a challenge for the program staff, with workers often dropping out after receiving training. Continually training new outreach workers has been costly and time consuming.
- *Social stigma.* Reliance faced initial challenges in its awareness and education programs because of the social stigma associated with HIV and AIDS and sexually transmitted infections. Workers hesitated to ask questions during training sessions, though they often returned to clear up misconceptions. And villagers were concerned about the proximity of the medical center to their homes, fearing that it could expose them to infections from visiting patients.
- *Monitoring and evaluation.* Reliance staff believe that monitoring and evaluation of the program need to be strengthened, with clearly defined targets established for evaluating all partners.

Other lessons learned

- *Financial sustainability.* The Gujarat State AIDS Control Society provides funds to LVS for its counseling, training, and dissemination services and for the cost of medicines. Thus the continued support of LVS as a program partner depends largely on the continued financial support of the Gujarat State AIDS Control Society.

Future plans

At the Hazira site, where Reliance has largely concentrated its efforts, the company has begun to construct a new center that can accommodate more patients. Future plans also call for replicating the program at other company sites. In addition, the company is considering implementing similar HIV and AIDS initiatives at Reliance gas stations on the highways, targeted to the trucking population. Given the plans to extend and expand the program, evaluating its impact to date and assessing the effectiveness of its interventions will be especially important.

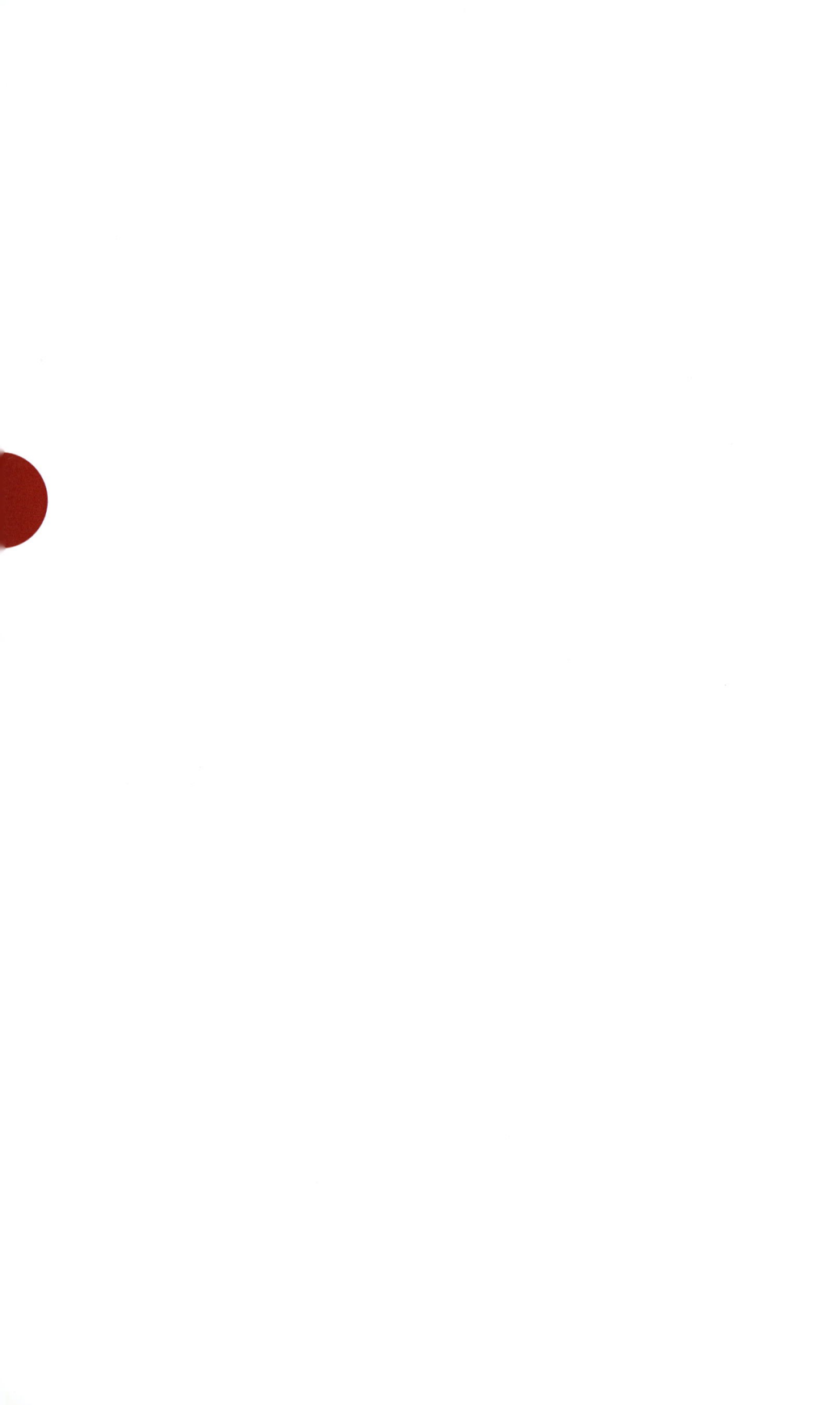

Case Study:
Transport Corporation of India Limited

Overview

Long-distance truckers have been found to be at high risk for HIV and other sexually transmitted infections.[9] Transport Corporation of India (TCI), as a major cargo transport company, recognized the importance of truckers in its business and launched a project specifically targeted to this population. This five-year HIV prevention project, Project Kavach (a Hindi word meaning *protection* or *shield*), is being implemented by TCI's social arm, the TCI Foundation, and by the Avahan India AIDS Initiative, which is funded by the Bill & Melinda Gates Foundation.

The project is a comprehensive, integrated approach to reducing the transmission of HIV and other sexually transmitted infections among long-distance truckers by:

- Providing diagnosis and treatment of sexually transmitted infections through project clinics.

---

9. The information in the TCI case study is based on personal interviews with TCI Foundation officials in Delhi and personnel responsible for implementing the program in Bangalore as well as internal documents shared by foundation staff during site visits in Delhi and Bangalore. The information is current as of September 2006.

33

- Using behavior change communication to encourage truckers to adopt safer sexual behavior and practices.
- Promoting condom use among the target population.

Because long-distance truckers are highly mobile, they need access to medical facilities where they travel. Project Kavach has therefore located its "Khushi" (a Hindi word for happiness) clinics at 17 major trucker halt points in nine Indian states. Each halt point sees about 20,000–30,000 truckers a year as they stop to rest and to repair their vehicles and the like.

These project sites were selected with the aim of reaching a target group of about 1.4 million long-distance truckers (drivers and crew members) nationwide through clinics, peer education, and condom distribution. To run the clinics and undertake other activities, the TCI Foundation has contracted with NGOs across the country.

Truckers' mobility also means that medical records are hard to maintain. The project deals with this challenge by issuing truckers a "Khushi passport"—a diary recording their medical history, diagnoses, and medications—that they can present at any project clinic.

The project has reached large numbers of truckers and others. Between January 2005 and March 2006 alone, its clinics treated nearly 43,000 people for sexually transmitted infections, 82 percent of them truckers. During the same period the project also distributed more than 700,000 condoms.[10]

Business background

Established in 1958, TCI is now among the leading conventional cargo transport companies in Asia. It transports cargo ranging from raw ma-

---

10. Condoms are also widely available along the truck routes through social marketing.

terials and agricultural and industrial products to consumer durables and drugs and pharmaceuticals. Recently TCI has started also transporting more sophisticated cargo, such as refrigerated, time-sensitive, and high-value items. The company's 4,000 trucker employees and fleet of more than 3,000 owned or contracted trucks move 4 million metric tons of goods annually. The company's annual turnover is Rs 1,000 crores (US$220 million).

Why do something about HIV and AIDS?

Studies show that long-distance truckers are at high risk for HIV and other sexually transmitted infections. Among India's 5–6 million truckers, nearly half work on long-distance routes across the country. Approximately 300,000 long-distance truckers in India are living with HIV.

HIV and AIDS interventions for truckers in India have been under state government programs, which lack oversight by a national program. Moreover, most government HIV and AIDS interventions have lacked strategic locations and adequate health services for this high-risk population.

> We have begun this program because we feel morally responsible for an important stakeholder: the trucker community. Our efforts will continue to address the HIV and AIDS epidemic.
>
> —D. P. Agarwal, Vice Chairman and Managing Director, TCI

To address this problem, the Bill & Melinda Gates Foundation launched the Avahan India AIDS Initiative, a large-scale HIV prevention program, in December 2003. This program focuses on the needs of several target groups: sex workers and their clients, men who have sex with men, long-distance truckers, and injecting drug users.

Asked by Avahan to participate in the program, TCI agreed, considering this an opportunity to reach out to one of its key stakeholders, the Indian trucking community.

The program

TCI's HIV program centers on Project Kavach. Launched in December 2003 and operated by TCI's social arm, the TCI Foundation, this five-year project is targeted to around 1.4 million long-distance truckers in nine states (about 30 percent of the country's trucking population and 60 percent of its long-distance truckers).[11]

The project is implemented through a chain of Khushi clinics at 17 high-volume transshipment hubs where truckers halt for at least 12 hours. Located along the Golden Quadrilateral—the 5,846-kilometer network of highways connecting Delhi, Kolkata, Chennai, and Mumbai—these clinics each serve an inflow of 100 truckers a day on average. The clinics also serve the local community, including workers employed at the halt points.

The program also uses some nontraditional outlets, such as tea shops, tobacco outlets, and roadside cafes and eateries, to distribute condoms. While interacting with truckers, shopkeepers at these outlets provide background information about HIV and AIDS and the dangers of not using condoms. The program enlists the services of truckers for peer education too. Both the shopkeepers and the truckers involved in peer education— referred to as secondary peer educators—offer their services voluntarily.

---

11. Initially the program targeted truckers through services at truck stops and halt points in 15 states. But in 2006 a strategic redesign narrowed the focus to an improved package of services delivered at high-volume truck stops where truckers spend significant time—transport hubs that link almost all major national highways in India. Clinics at halt points with smaller inflows of truckers were closed.

Interventions for truckers

Project Kavach has four main components:

- Clinical management of sexually transmitted infections and related counseling.
- Behavior change communication.
- Condom promotion and social marketing.
- Community mobilization.

Because management of sexually transmitted infections is considered an important factor in stemming the spread of HIV, STI treatment and counseling have been a vital part of Project Kavach. To provide such services, the clinics are staffed by 80 qualified doctors, nurses, and counselors (picture 1).

Other project efforts are designed around truckers' activities. During their halts truckers receive orders and payments, service their vehicles, and transact business with contractors and brokers (agents who book vehicles). The project uses the spare time that truckers have left to share information and educate them on such topics as the risks of unprotected sex and the advantages of using condoms.

The Khushi clinics are also equipped to treat general ailments, since trucking hubs, located along stretches of highway outside cities, lack basic medical facilities. Positioning Khushi clinics as general health and STI treatment centers has the added advantage of reducing any hesitance truckers may feel about entering a clinic.

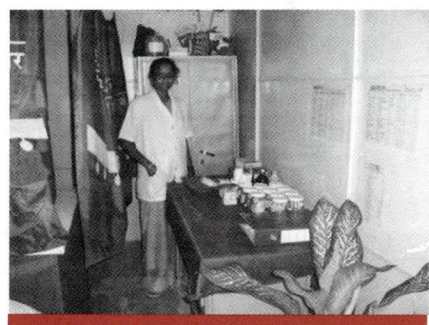

Picture 1. Medical officer at a Khushi clinic

Other features of the project are also designed to fit the circumstances of truckers, including their mobility.

Innovations for medical tracking

A trucker making a first visit to a clinic is issued a "Khushi passport," a diary recording details of the trucker's medical history and the diagnosis and any medication given during that visit. The trucker is expected to bring this diary each time he visits a clinic. The diary also contains the addresses of all 17 Khushi clinics in India to encourage the trucker to use their services when traveling in the area where they are located.

Each trucker visiting a clinic also has a unique identification number, which helps clinic staff track his medical records in their database. This central database is maintained by the TCI Foundation's national project management unit in Gurgaon, Delhi, which collects the data from each Khushi clinic. The management information system not only allows access to medical records, it also supports analysis providing useful insights into the prevalence of HIV and other sexually transmitted infections and helps in the annual monitoring and evaluation of the program.

Treatment and services

Each Khushi clinic follows comprehensive clinical operating procedures that were designed by Family Health International and the WHO, based on Indian clinical guidance where available.

While registration and consultation at the clinics are free, truckers are required to pay for medicines (priced at cost) to encourage them to take the treatment more seriously. During the consultation each trucker is also counseled on basic facts about sexual health and safety.

Khushi clinics do not have laboratory services, instead relying on their referral system for these. The project has established links with government laboratories to provide syphilis testing (rapid plasma reagin and Venereal Disease Research Laboratory screening). Rapid HIV testing is conducted at only one project site, that in Neelamangala, Bangalore.

Setup and operation of the clinics

Setting up Khushi clinics involved a number of steps. The TCI Foundation first had to research trucker long-halt points to identify strategic locations for clinics. At the same time it also had to identify, for each site, a local NGO that had the capacity and willingness to be responsible for a Khushi clinic and carry out behavior change communication. In addition, the foundation had to seek permission from the local State AIDS Control Society to operate in the area. This step was important so as to avoid duplicating interventions, since several halt points have more than one NGO operating through various targeted HIV and AIDS programs.

Operation of each clinic has been contracted to an NGO with responsibility for running the clinic, disseminating information, providing referrals, and the like (table 2). The clinic staff, comprising outreach workers, doctors, and nurses, are all full-time employees of these NGOs. The TCI Foundation provides the NGOs the funds to run the clinics. With its national team of 33 professionals, the foundation supervises the work of the NGOs to ensure that they are complying with the minimum standards set for all NGOs participating in the program for truckers.

In addition to a static Khushi clinic that serves as the hub of project activities at each halt point, there are tents, mobile vans, and clinics in the premises of brokers and local transporters (picture 2). These satellites were established because a transshipment hub or halt point covers a large area and cannot reach all truckers.

Table 2. Khushi clinics in India			
Region and clinic	*NH*	*NGO operating the clinic*	*State*
Bangalore			
Neelamangala DTT	4	Bhoruka Charitable Trust	Karnataka
Hyderabad Autonagar	7 & 8	Bhoruka Charitable Trust	Andhra Pradesh
Icchapuram	5	BPWT	Andhra Pradesh
Hubli-Dharwad	4	Bhoruka Charitable Trust	Karnataka
Jamsola	6	Bhoruka Charitable Trust	Orissa
Delhi			
Delhi SGTN	1	Child Survival India	Delhi
Delhi UP Border	2	CEVA	Uttar Pradesh
Kanpur	2	Nirman Seva Sanstha	Uttar Pradesh
Jaipur VIA with JK satellite at intersection at Transport Nagar	8	VATSALYA	Rajasthan
Agra	2	CREATE	Uttar Pradesh
Varanasi	2	Jankalyan Maha Samiti	Uttar Pradesh
Nagpur			
Mumbai Kalamboli	4	Bombay Leprosy Project	Maharashtra
Indore	3	Bhartiya Gramin Mahila Sangh	Madhya Pradesh
Pune Nigdi	4	Seva Dham Trust	Maharashtra
Nagpur Pardi with satellite at Wadi	6	Indian Institute of Youth Welfare	Maharashtra
Jamshedpur	33	TSRDS	Jharkand
Dhanbad	2 & 23	Gram Pradyogik Vikas Sanstha	Jharkand

Note: NH is national highway number.
Source: TCI Foundation.

Interventions for the community

Besides providing services to truckers, the NGO staff at each site also reaches out to the community and educates the local populace about HIV and AIDS. These activities have been particularly helpful in addressing the social stigma and discrimination associated with HIV and AIDS. The development of interpersonal relations tools customized for the different target groups has helped in making these awareness activities effective.

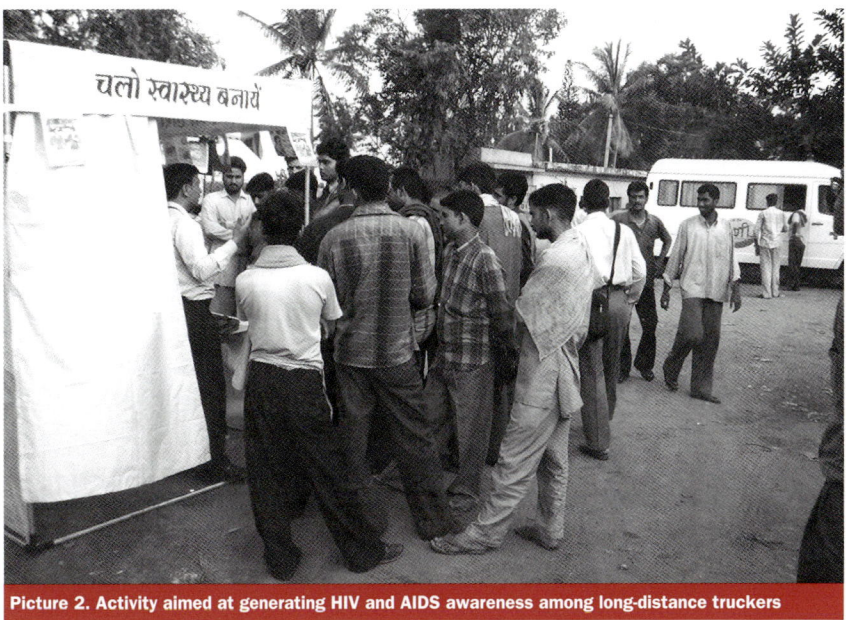

Picture 2. Activity aimed at generating HIV and AIDS awareness among long-distance truckers

Internal workplace program

After launching Project Kavach, TCI began to develop its own workplace policy on HIV and AIDS, with support from the ILO, Delhi. In 2004 the company initiated an HIV program for its workplace. It has begun to create a cadre of peer educators who will share HIV and AIDS information with their colleagues at the workplace and distribute information, education, and communication materials. The company would like to eventually reach out to all 4,000 employees.

In addition to its awareness program, the company is funding the cost of antiretroviral therapy for two to three employees.

Partnerships

Project Kavach depends on a range of partnerships. The program draws expertise not only from the partner NGOs operating the clinics but also from other Avahan partners: Program for Appropriate Technology in Health (PATH) for effective communication campaigns, Population Services International (PSI) for social marketing of condoms, Family Health International (FHI) for medical training, and CARE for community involvement (figure 3). Each of these provides their services in the transshipment hubs serving the trucking population. The TCI Foundation provides infrastructure such as office space and equipment

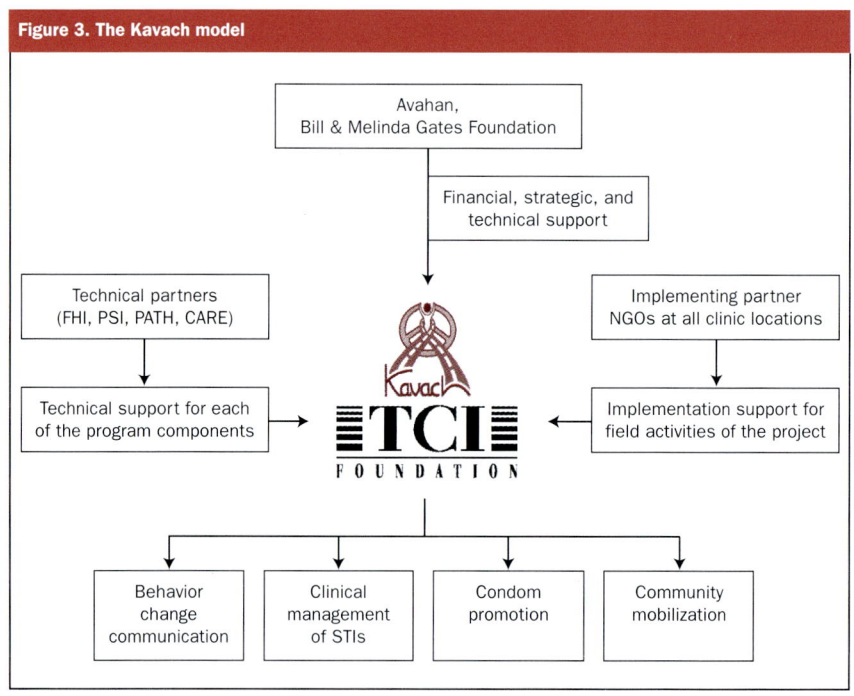

Figure 3. The Kavach model

through its regional offices (Pune and Bangalore). And Avahan provides funding for medicines and for staff salaries (for the TCI Foundation and partners).

As noted, the TCI Foundation supervises the work of the partner NGOs to ensure quality of implementation and efficiency of service. The foundation's staff is also responsible for networking and coordinating the program with the other Avahan partners.

The project has worked to build the capacity of the NGOs through training programs to ensure that these organizations can continue the fight against HIV and AIDS even after the project ends. To further decentralize the program, steering committees made up of local brokers, truck owners, and truckers are being set up to form important nodal points for projects in the local communities.

Funding

Avahan of the Bill & Melinda Gates Foundation is providing US$8 million for the five-year program. The TCI Foundation is exploring a strategy for ensuring that the program can be self-sustaining after 2008.

Outreach

The project's outreach—through communication, condom marketing, and treatment—involves impressive numbers. Consider the achievements of the project's team of 197 outreach workers and 942 secondary peer educators:

- On average the team has made 63,000 effective contacts monthly through one-on-one and group discussions.

- By March 2006 the team had made more than one million contacts with truckers alone.

The project's condom marketing efforts have been extensive:

- The project has set up 979 nontraditional condom outlets nationwide.
- Between January 2005 and March 2006 outreach workers, condom outlets, clinics, and peer educators distributed 706,250 condoms.

The record of treatment provided by clinics is similarly impressive. Between January 2005 and March 2006:

- Clinics provided treatment of sexually transmitted infections for 4,000 people a month on average, and for a total of 42,906 people. Of these, 35,059 (82 percent) were truckers. The rest were local shopkeepers, mechanics, vendors, and others in the local population.
- Clinics provided treatment of general ailments for 9,000 people a month on average, and for a total of 92,053. Of these, 64,488 (70 percent) were truckers.

Lessons learned

The TCI Foundation monitors Project Kavach by periodically meeting with its partner NGOs to discuss the progress of their interventions and areas of possible improvement. This regular monitoring, considered one of the strengths of the program, has identified useful lessons.

Key success factors

- *Wide network of implementing partners.* The TCI Foundation's success in implementing the HIV program on such a large scale is due largely to the network of NGOs that form the backbone of the project. Besides outreach, this network provides the program with technical support and local knowledge.
- *Location of clinics.* The location of the clinics along highways not only helps fill the gap in medical services for truckers, it also leads to a big inflow of patients, which has helped the program acquire a national reputation.
- *Diverse expertise from other Avahan partners.* Project Kavach has been able to take a holistic approach to delivering services because it can draw on the diverse expertise of other Avahan partners.

Key challenges

- *Sensitizing other industry stakeholders.* TCI has been seeking partnerships with other companies that also interact with the trucking industry on a large scale, including oil and gas companies with gas stations along the highways. But it has found that many companies have not yet realized the enormity of the HIV and AIDS problem, its repercussions, and the high cost of inaction. The company is therefore conducting advocacy efforts through industry bodies and with individual companies to sensitize businesses to the issue.
- *Behavioral change.* Truckers repeatedly exposed to the same information experience message fatigue. In addition, repeated interventions targeted at the trucking community have resulted in negative branding, stigmatizing truckers as people who practice

unsafe sexual behavior. The program is therefore devising new forms of communication to increase its acceptability to the trucking community. One innovation, Magnet Theater, involves truckers themselves as the protagonists in theater performances. In addition, the TCI Foundation has found that efforts to change behavior may not be entirely successful unless they simultaneously address such factors as harsh working conditions and exposure to a high-risk environment.

Other lessons learned

- *Payment as a way to create ownership.* A key lesson from the program is that when truckers pay for their medication, they develop a sense of ownership for the entire treatment process and take their treatment more seriously.
- *Importance of easy access to services.* The TCI Foundation observed that truckers rarely leave their halt points to go into the city to use medical facilities. Khushi clinics, located at trucker halt points, have been successful because they provide easy access.
- *Myths about HIV and AIDS.* Many myths and misconceptions about the spread of HIV persist, leading to unsafe behavior among truckers. For example, many truckers practiced unsafe sex with their male cotravelers because they believed that HIV does not spread through sex with men. The program has therefore focused on addressing misconceptions through its information, education, and communication material and sessions.

Future plans

The TCI Foundation is exploring several plans and ideas for making Project Kavach more effective:

- Strengthening links with testing and treatment facilities around each clinic so as to develop a strong referral network.
- Enabling each Khushi clinic to undertake HIV testing.
- Building a mechanism to track truckers' movements. The project now has no way of ensuring that truckers needing further treatment would return to a clinic (and truckers often lose their Khushi passports).
- Documenting the lessons and achievements of the program to help in developing a future strategy.

As part of the efforts to make the project more effective, it will be important for the TCI Foundation to evaluate the project's impact and the cost and effectiveness of its interventions.

Case Study:
Delhi Metro Rail Corporation Limited

Overview

Building the metro rail system in Delhi has been a massive construction project drawing workers from across India.[12] Migrant workers typically are especially at risk for HIV, as a study focusing on the project's workforce confirmed. To help reduce the risk of HIV among this population, Delhi Metro Rail Corporation (DMRC), the public sector company responsible for constructing, operating, and maintaining the metro rail system, initiated an HIV and AIDS program targeted to the laborers working on one of the metro lines.

The program focused mainly on increasing HIV and AIDS awareness and promoting the use of condoms. Lacking the technical capacity to carry out the program, DMRC contracted with an NGO, Modicare Foundation, to do so. The program, originally planned to run from January through June 2005, was extended through September 2005 and covered more than 3,000 workers.

12. The information in the DMRC case study is based on responses by DMRC and Modicare Foundation to questions sent to them by email; personal interviews and interactions with the DMRC official responsible for implementing the program and with Modicare Foundation officials; and a project report by Modicare Foundation (2006). The information is current as of September 2006.

49

DMRC has used its influence over contractors to further its goals in combating HIV and AIDS: the contracts it signs with these companies now require that they carry out HIV prevention and control activities for employees working on DMRC projects. DMRC has developed an HIV and AIDS policy to guide contractors in implementing these programs.

Business background

DMRC was formed in May 1995 by the national and Delhi state governments to provide a rail-based transport system that will alleviate Delhi's ever growing transport congestion and vehicular pollution. The government of Japan has contributed more than half the cost of this project, through a soft loan disbursed by DMRC's major funding agency, the Japan Bank for International Cooperation (JBIC).

Delhi's metro rail system, to be constructed in four phases covering 245 kilometers, is scheduled to be finished in 2021. Today three functioning lines connect central Delhi to east, north, and southwest Delhi.

DMRC is responsible not only for construction of the system but also for its operation and maintenance. It has 450 personnel in its construction department and 3,000 staff for system operation and maintenance. Supply chain partners provide critical support, including labor, machinery and components, and maintenance services.

Why do something about HIV and AIDS?

The impetus for DMRC's HIV and AIDS program came from a study commissioned by JBIC in accordance with its guidelines for approving loans and investments.[13] Conducted by the Voluntary Health Association

13. In approving loans and investments, JBIC is required by its guidelines to examine such issues as impact on indigenous peoples and their heritage, gender issues, children's

of India, the study assessed the vulnerability to HIV of the workforce on one line of phase 1 of the Delhi Metro project (VHAI 2003). The study produced disturbing findings:

- In the sample of 1,000 workers surveyed, 59.3 percent had little or no knowledge about HIV and AIDS.
- Around 86.4 percent had little or no knowledge about how HIV is transmitted.
- The practice of using condoms to prevent transmission of HIV was unknown.
- Around 80–90 percent of the workers had a negative attitude toward people living with HIV and AIDS.
- Respondents reported visits to sex workers.

The study highlighted the predominance of migrant workers in the workforce on the Delhi Metro project and the vulnerability of this population to HIV. According to a project document (Modicare Foundation 2006), around 15,000 workers have participated in the Delhi Metro project, a substantial number of them migrant workers from other Indian states—Bihar, Chhattisgarh, Madhya Pradesh, Orissa, Rajasthan, and West Bengal. These migrant workers face conditions that can encourage high-risk sexual behavior: separation from family, alienation from sociocultural norms, loneliness, and a sense of anonymity that offers greater sexual freedom. In addition, the workers are uneducated, live in unhygienic, often crowded quarters, and are unaware of safe health practices. All these factors increase their vulnerability to communicable diseases such as tuberculosis and also to HIV.

Based on this study, DMRC decided to initiate an HIV and AIDS program and fund it entirely through its own resources. JBIC helped in

---

rights, and HIV and AIDS. JBIC also actively encourages the mitigation of adverse social impacts and promotes social participation for certain projects. See JBIC (2005).

> Our program is a proactive step to safeguard our workers and also uphold our social responsibility as corporate citizens.
>
> —C. B. K. Rao, Director,
> Delhi Metro Rail Corporation

creating a strategy for the program through appropriately defined objectives, action plans, and time frame.

The program

The program initiated by DMRC was aimed at preventing HIV by promoting awareness and improved sexual behavior, attitudes, and practices among migrant workers on the Delhi Metro project. Recognizing that it lacked the technical capacity to implement the program, DMRC used a bidding process to recruit the services of an organization with the technical expertise needed. This led to the selection of Modicare Foundation, a well-respected NGO with experience in carrying out HIV and AIDS programs, as the implementing partner.

To extend program activities to future DMRC projects, the company developed an HIV and AIDS policy with expectations for contractors engaged in those projects (box 1).

Awareness and prevention activities at the workplace

The program's target group initially was around 2,000 migrant workers who were employed by DMRC's contractors on the site for phase 1, specifically those working on line 3 from central to southwest Delhi. But when DMRC extended the program by three months, through September 2005, it expanded the target group by 1,000.

Modicare profiled the target group as follows:

Box 1. An HIV and AIDS workplace policy to guide future programs

To provide clear guidelines for HIV and AIDS programs implemented in future projects, DMRC developed the "Workplace Policy on HIV/AIDS Prevention & Control for Workmen Engaged by Contractors," based on the International Labour Organization's code of practice on HIV and AIDS. The policy expects DMRC contractors:

- To create awareness about HIV and AIDS among their workers.
- To build institutional capacity for HIV and AIDS programs through training.
- To establish links for diagnosis and treatment of affected workers; for monitoring, implementation, and documentation of program activities; for peer education; and for social marketing of condoms.

DMRC established this policy only after soliciting inputs from its contractors and checking with them on the policy's feasibility. The company also took into account its own experience in implementing projects. The process was facilitated by Modicare Foundation.

DMRC has incorporated the policy into the contract it signs with its contractors and suppliers. The agreement also expects contractors to extend organizational support to the HIV and AIDS program and identify peer educators. When peer educators who have been trained as part of the program leave a contractor's employment, the contractor has to identify and train a replacement.

- The age group of the workers was 20–45.
- Two-thirds were married men, living away from their families.
- The workers lived in makeshift rooms at the construction sites or in rented accommodations in nearby slums.
- Even small rooms were usually shared by 10–15 people.

The program had four main components aimed at HIV and AIDS awareness and prevention:

- Advocacy.
- Institutional capacity building.
- Peer education.
- Condom promotion.

Advocacy

The advocacy efforts began by developing information, education, and communication material suited to the program. This included posters, pamphlets, calendars with messages on HIV and AIDS, and lists of STI clinics, voluntary counseling and testing centers, and outlets distributing condoms. Some posters were developed by Modicare Foundation; others were brought in from the National AIDS Control Organization and other sources (picture 3).

In addition, activities sought to generate awareness among workers in the target group using the behavior change communication model. Modicare developed modules for its facilitators to use in sharing information on HIV and AIDS within groups of 15–20 workers.

Institutional capacity building

To help ensure effective implementation, the program set up a technical advisory committee—formed of representatives from DMRC, JBIC, the ILO, and Modicare—to provide technical support and to monitor the program. It also held an orientation session for DMRC safety managers, safety officers, and engineers and for project managers of construction companies working for DMRC. This was intended to sensitize them to issues relating to HIV and AIDS as well as to ensure their participation and cooperation in future program activities.

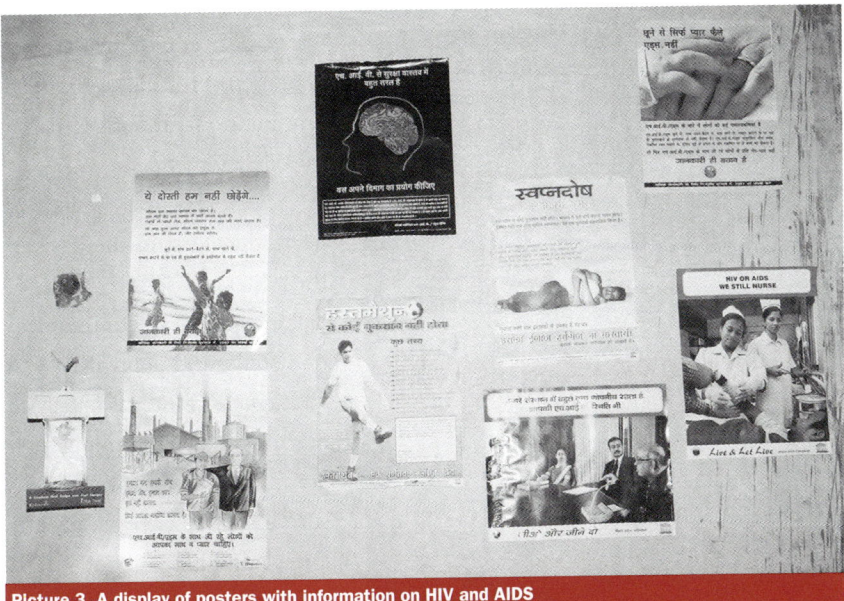

Picture 3. A display of posters with information on HIV and AIDS

To help overcome the lack of its own medical facilities, the program worked to develop links with STI clinics and voluntary counseling and testing centers—critical for a successful HIV prevention program. The program succeeded in establishing links with 13 government hospitals close to Delhi Metro project sites where it could encourage the target group to obtain treatment and counseling.

Peer education

The program used peer education to encourage the flow of information on HIV and AIDS and related issues from informed workers to their colleagues. Informal communication has been found to create greater acceptance of information than more formal ways of communication. The

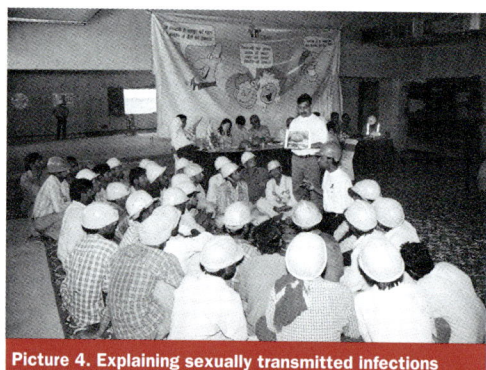

Picture 4. Explaining sexually transmitted infections using pictorial flashcards

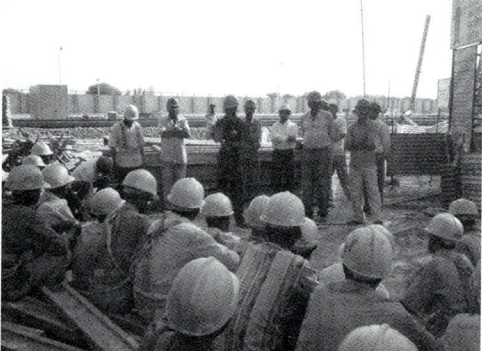

Picture 5. A peer educator during a session at a construction site

use of peer education was also aimed at creating a nondiscriminatory and nonstigmatizing environment.

The program identified peer educators on the basis of their literacy, sensitivity, leadership qualities, communication skills, and popularity with colleagues. Modicare carried out an intensive training program for peer educators to ensure that they were sufficiently knowledgeable about HIV transmission and prevention and equipped to address issues related to sexual health. It also gave each one a kit containing material on HIV and other sexually transmitted infections and condoms for demonstration and distribution.

Peer educators were asked to reach out to their colleagues through both one-on-one and group discussions, addressing queries about HIV and other sexually transmitted infections (picture 4), encouraging safe sexual behavior by promoting and distributing condoms, and distributing information, education, and communication material. Peer educators also referred people to STI clinics and voluntary counseling and testing centers. Settings for peer education sessions included the construction site (picture 5).

Condom promotion

Promoting the correct and consistent use of condoms as an essential factor in preventing HIV and other sexually transmitted infections was an important part of the program. The program found that distributing condoms was a major factor in increasing the demand for them and resulted in correct and habitual use by the members of the target group. Some 90 percent of the workers covered by Modicare, and 67 percent of those covered by the peer educators, accessed condoms.

> During one of my sessions a boy shared with me that he had been suffering from an STI and that he had had sex with an unknown woman a few months back. On my advice he underwent [HIV] testing and was found to be negative. He took treatment for STI and is leading a normal life, free of infection now.
>
> —Mahesh Kumar, peer educator

Project monitoring, reporting, and documentation

The program put into place a systematic monitoring plan, under the technical advisory committee, to track implementation. Modicare Foundation used forms soliciting feedback from its facilitators to assess effectiveness. Monthly reports consolidated information on activities conducted, including street plays and informal sessions by peer educators. Peer educators and Modicare Foundation coordinators and facilitators met regularly. Periodic meetings were also held between DMRC officials, the technical advisory committee, and the project team leader from Modicare Foundation.

Funding

The program budget was close to Rs 6.5 lakhs (US$14,500), funded entirely from DMRC's own resources.

Outreach

The program reached 3,270 workers, exceeding the target of 3,000 (table 3). In addition, nearly 3,000 workers obtained condoms from Modicare.

Following up with workers contacted as part of the program proved difficult, since the workers changed jobs often. But Modicare Foundation conducted follow-up discussions with 10 percent of the workers to assess their information recall after their initial information session with a facilitator, usually 10–15 days after that session.

Results of this follow-up, based on 308 questionnaires, showed that:

- About half the workers questioned recalled three modes of HIV transmission, and more than a third recalled two (figure 4).
- Almost all the workers recalled use of a condom as a method for preventing transmission of HIV (figure 5).

Table 3. Outreach indicators for DMRC program, January–September 2005

Item	Number
Workers covered	3,270
Peer educators trained	47
Metro stations covered	29
Construction companies covered	13
Street plays and puppet shows arranged	48
Magic shows arranged	27
Condom demonstrations held	229
Persons obtaining condoms from Modicare Foundation	2,946

Source: Modicare Foundation, 2006.

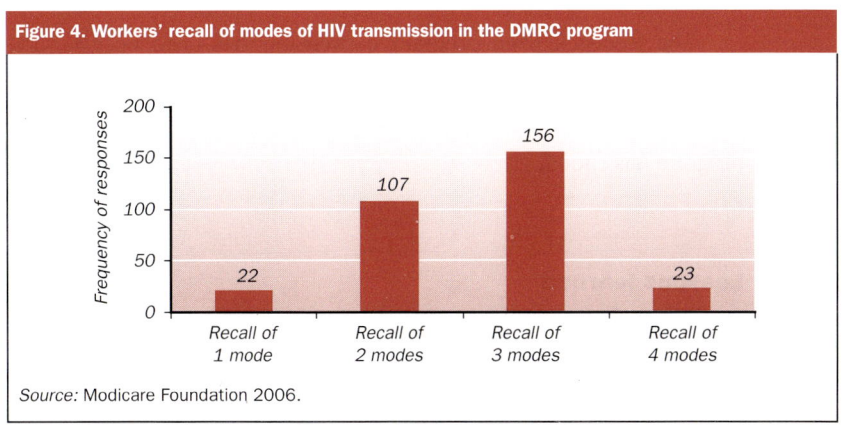

Figure 4. Workers' recall of modes of HIV transmission in the DMRC program

Source: Modicare Foundation 2006.

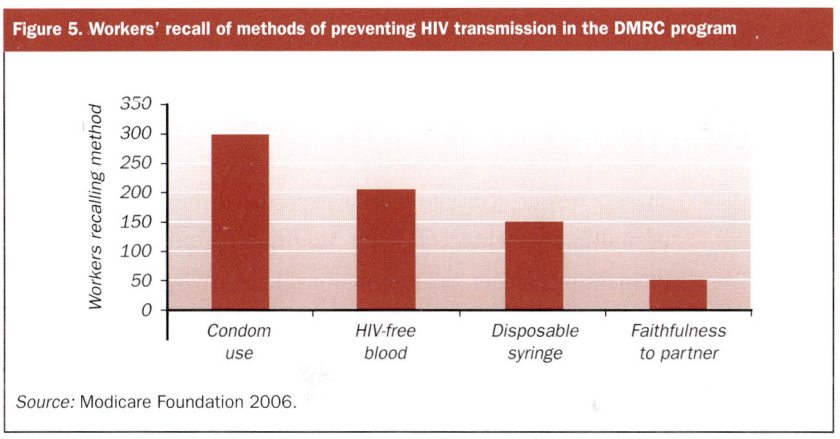

Figure 5. Workers' recall of methods of preventing HIV transmission in the DMRC program

Source: Modicare Foundation 2006.

Even more important, the sessions led to changes in behavior among the workers:

- Some 25 percent (78 out of 308) reported using condoms after sessions.
- Referrals and visits to HIV and STI clinics increased.
- Some peer educators reported changing their own formerly high-risk behavior and attitudes after being sensitized by peer educator training.

The feedback from program participants has been positive. The workers have expressed a desire for the program to be continued, and the peer educators continue to counsel their colleagues even though the program has ended.

Lessons learned

The program identified several success factors, challenges, and other lessons based on its results.

Key success factors

- *Partnership of multiple stakeholders.* A key factor in the program's success was its access to diverse expertise through a partnership of multiple stakeholders—with Modicare Foundation as the implementing partner, the International Labour Organization as the technical adviser, and the Japan Bank for International Cooperation as a strategy adviser.
- *Peer education.* Involving peer educators helped both expand outreach and establish contact with sex workers, who were persuaded to keep condoms for clients. Around 20 percent of the peer educators are still active and have been in regular touch with Modicare Foundation.
- *Cooperation from contractors.* The special effort made to sensitize the contractors to the issues was key in gaining their support for the program. Contractors even gave their workers time off to participate in the meetings on issues relating to HIV and AIDS.
- *Informal outreach to workers.* Using informal means to reach out to migrant workers—such as meeting them on their home ground

or using their dialect when conversing with them—made the workers feel comfortable and helped immensely in achieving the targets.

Key challenges

- *Poor access to health services.* With government medical and testing facilities unavailable on weekends, laborers often ended up going to fake doctors. Good health services, including mobile health facilities, need to be made more accessible to the workers.
- *Mobility of workers.* The high mobility of workers made it difficult for Modicare Foundation to follow up with the target group after the initial information session. Even so, the agency achieved a follow-up rate of 10 percent. The high mobility also created a challenge for peer education: trained peer educators could leave their jobs, and training replacements was costly. To help strengthen and stabilize the peer education system, DMRC has incorporated a clause into its agreement with contractors and suppliers requiring that they identify a peer educator likely to stay for a long time. If a peer educator leaves a contractor, the contractor has to get a replacement trained at its own cost.
- *Access to condoms.* The unpredictability of workers' job locations made getting condoms to the workers a challenge. Modicare Foundation suggests that DMRC could work with Hindustan Latex Limited (an Indian government enterprise) or another manufacturer of condoms to provide condom vending machines at selected sites. These machines could be kept under the custody of the contractor in charge of the construction site. Alternatively, DMRC could rely on peer educators and nontraditional outlets such as tea and cigarette vendors to distribute condoms.

Other lessons learned

- *Importance of links with health services.* DMRC found that creating links with existing health services is important: it enables the target group to gain access to services not provided by the program and also avoids duplicating services.
- *Programs for all cadres of employees.* Modicare Foundation believes that HIV and AIDS programs should cover all cadres of employees, not just contract workers. Awareness among senior employees will ensure that they appreciate the need for such programs, support activities, encourage peer educators, and help create a nonthreatening environment for dealing with HIV and AIDS. And greater awareness among all workers will reduce the stigma associated with HIV and AIDS.
- *Importance of monitoring and evaluation.* The program's monitoring system was an important feature, allowing the company to track progress in implementation and assess the program's effectiveness.

Future plans

DMRC plans to implement a similar program in the next phase of the Delhi Metro construction, identifying a new implementing partner for this program. The company's HIV and AIDS policy for contract workers, to be implemented in this next phase of construction, is further evidence that DMRC has taken the risks posed by HIV and AIDS to this population seriously.

Case Study:
DCM Shriram Consolidated Limited

Overview

DCM Shriram Consolidated Limited (DSCL), a company with interests mainly in chemicals and agribusiness, operates in western and northern India.[14] The western state of Rajasthan is home to the company's main manufacturing plant, in Kota, which has also been the site of its HIV and AIDS program. The program is uniquely local, drawing on local culture and adapting information, education, and communication material to appeal to local sensibilities.

Committed to providing a safe and healthy working environment, the company holds regular group sessions to build HIV and AIDS awareness among its employees. DSCL's occupational health doctor speaks on the basics of HIV and AIDS awareness and prevention. But then follows a song or poem in the local dialect to convey messages more light-heartedly. The company also uses cultural performances at festivals or other important events at the Kota plant to generate mass awareness.

---

14. The information in the DSCL case study is based on DSCL's response to a questionnaire sent to the company by email; personal interviews with the company's chief executive officer and with the officials responsible for implementing the program; and a site visit. The information is current as of September 2006.

Communicating messages in ways that fit the local culture and local sensibilities has helped the program capture the attention of the target audience. It has also helped the program gain acceptance among the local population.

Business background

DSCL has diverse business interests ranging from agribusiness (sugar, fertilizers, agri-retail) to chemicals (chlorine, caustic soda), plastics (PVC resins, polymer compounds), and others (cement, textiles, energy services, real estate development). The corporate office is in New Delhi, and the main manufacturing plant in Kota, in the western state of Rajasthan.

The Kota plant, the site of the company's HIV and AIDS intervention, houses manufacturing facilities for fertilizers, plastics, chlor alkali, and cement as well as a captive power plant. This site has 1,600 full-time employees, 1,500 daily contract workers, and 500 staff for security, manual labor, and the like.

The company's annual sales are Rs 23 billion (around US$500 million). DSCL's main supply chain partners—public enterprises and small and medium-size suppliers—provide raw materials such as coal, salt, naphtha, and limestone.

Why do something about HIV and AIDS?

DSCL's decision to initiate an HIV and AIDS program was motivated largely by its belief that AIDS is a public health challenge that could affect its workforce, its supply chain, its value chain partners, and the broader community. Looking at the experience of other countries, the company recognized that the business community, particularly in manufacturing,

Box 2. An HIV and AIDS policy shaped by many actors

DSCL's policy on HIV and AIDS focuses on providing a safe and healthy work environment, educating employees, and ensuring confidentiality and nondiscrimination. Adapted from the policy statement circulated by the Confederation of Indian Industry, the policy was shaped through detailed discussions held at various levels of the organization, including with employees, trade unions, and management.

needed to contribute to the fight against HIV and AIDS. Thus while no HIV-positive cases have yet been reported at the company's sites, advocacy efforts by industry associations in India convinced senior management that DSCL, as a responsible corporate citizen, needed to take part.

The company has adopted an HIV and AIDS policy out of a belief that the policy could serve as a key driver in initiating intervention programs (box 2).

The program

DSCL identified two potential target groups for its program: Its own steadily growing employee base, a large captive audience that could be informed about HIV and AIDS at the workplace and the large number of truckers who came to its factories (particularly in the sugar division, where many truckers offloaded sugarcane).

At an initial meeting to allocate responsibility for the program, DSCL decided to assign the program to an official who volunteered his efforts. The human resources unit normally would have led the program. But the official's demonstrated eagerness to be involved in an HIV program made him a promising choice.

The program began in January 2005 by gathering information about the issue, identifying resources such as organizations providing technical services, and developing information, education, and communication material. As many programs have done, DSCL's has created pamphlets containing information about HIV and AIDS, but much of its material shows unusual innovation. Cassettes intersperse HIV and AIDS messages with popular Hindi film songs. And songs are written in the local dialect to appeal to the diverse community working in the plant and living around it.

Awareness and prevention activities at the workplace

The company's awareness activities at the workplace center on group meetings where the occupational health team shares information about HIV and AIDS with DSCL employees. Sessions take place on the shop floor or near the factory entrance (picture 6). Meetings usually consist of a talk by the company's medical officer, messages on HIV and AIDS conveyed through poems, songs, or jokes in the local dialect, and a quiz to see whether participants have grasped the information. Sessions end with distribution of free condoms.

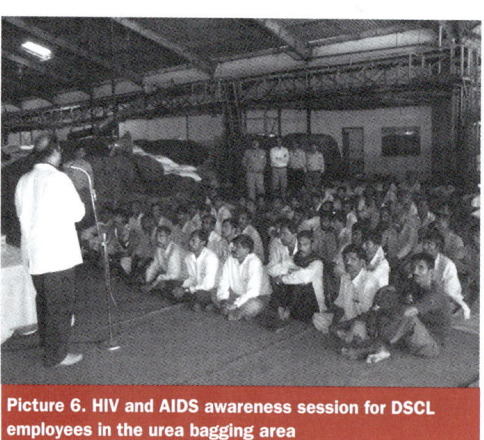

Picture 6. HIV and AIDS awareness session for DSCL employees in the urea bagging area

To encourage its contract employees to participate, the company sought the cooperation of the contractors in conducting the awareness sessions. Contract employees are more willing to spend time at these sessions if their employers are agreeable.

Outside the meetings, the occupational health team disseminates information about

HIV and AIDS to employees and workers through pamphlets, posters, and billboards created in-house. Some posters call out to the target audience to join the fight against HIV and AIDS (picture 7). Others quote a powerful speech by Nelson Mandela portraying HIV and AIDS as everyone's responsibility (picture 8). Awareness material is placed in prominent locations at the plant, such as in the visitors' lobby and on the notice board.

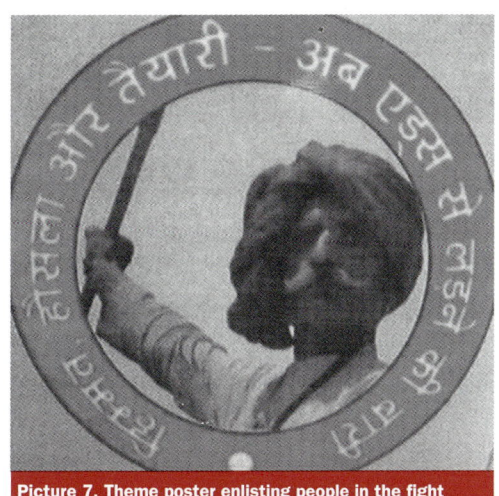

Picture 7. Theme poster enlisting people in the fight against HIV and AIDS

DSCL has made good use of the company's own resources in communicating information. For example, employees skilled in music, drama, writing, and poetry use their arts to convey messages about HIV and AIDS. One such employee, a talented singer and poet as well as a brilliant orator in the local dialect, accompanies DSCL's chief medical officer

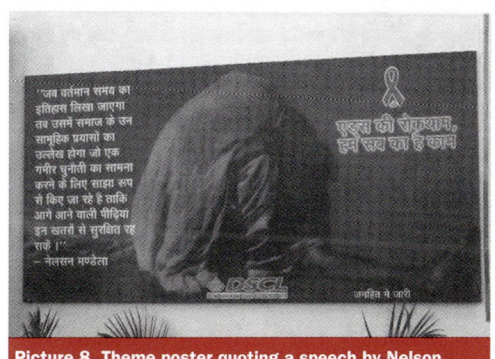

Picture 8. Theme poster quoting a speech by Nelson Mandela

to awareness sessions. These artists also convey messages during performances at interdepartmental cultural competitions, plant days, and other festive occasions.

The company disseminates information in other innovative ways as well. Its visitors' passes now include HIV and AIDS messages (picture 9). Films, plays, and cultural performances impart HIV and AIDS awareness

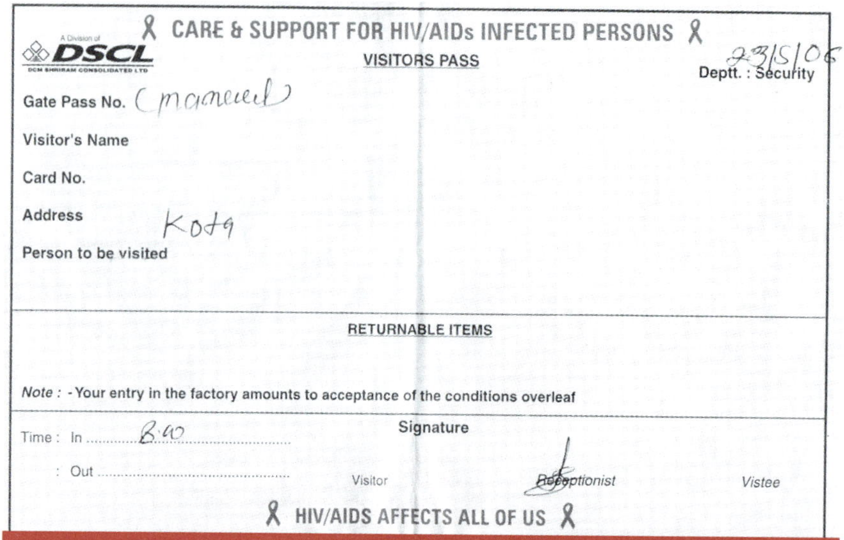

A Division of DSCL
DCM SHRIRAM CONSOLIDATED LTD

CARE & SUPPORT FOR HIV/AIDs INFECTED PERSONS

VISITORS PASS

Deptt. : Security 23/5/06

Gate Pass No. (manual)

Visitor's Name

Card No.

Address Kota

Person to be visited

RETURNABLE ITEMS

Note : - Your entry in the factory amounts to acceptance of the conditions overleaf

Time : In 8.40

: Out

Signature

Visitor *Receptionist* *Vistee*

HIV/AIDS AFFECTS ALL OF US

Picture 9. DSCL visitor's pass with HIV and AIDS messages

at public functions held to commemorate important company days or religious festivals. Films are screened occasionally in the canteens while the workers gather to eat. Films on HIV and AIDS are also shown to officers trained at the company's training institute.

For more informal communication with employees about HIV and AIDS, DSCL relies on its welfare officers. These officers, each responsible for the well-being of a certain number of employees, act as conduits between management and workers and as support systems and confidants for employees and their families. Their deep engagement with employees makes them well placed to spread awareness about HIV and AIDS and to provide individual counseling. The medical doctors in the plant and trained polyclinic staff also provide counseling.

DSCL does not have its own medical facilities for HIV and AIDS. But the city of Kota has a government-established blood testing and detection center. And DSCL's medical staff has received specialized training on HIV and AIDS, on such issues as primary care, visual diagnosis and management of opportunistic infections, lab diagnosis, and antiretroviral therapy. The staff conducts regular medical checkups on employees and is trained to notice symptomatic indicators of HIV and AIDS.

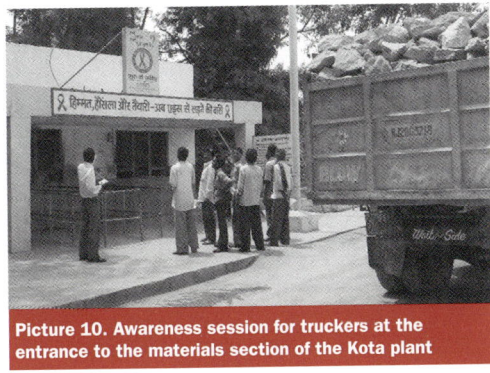

Picture 10. Awareness session for truckers at the entrance to the materials section of the Kota plant

While DSCL reports having no HIV-positive employees, it can arrange for antiretroviral therapy at the Kota government hospital. The company now covers the cost of treatment for some AIDS patients in the city of Kota even though they are not DSCL employees.

Interventions for the community

DSCL also conducts awareness sessions beyond the shop floor, for truckers who transport material to and from the company. The method is the same as that for employees: in a group session the company doctor shares information on HIV and AIDS, and then free condoms are distributed. The sessions for the truckers take place while their goods are being loaded or unloaded (picture 10).

DSCL has sometimes faced challenges in implementing its HIV and AIDS program while managing the varying expectations of the local community. But the company plans to reach out to the wider community through similar programs for local slum dwellers and drug addicts and through programs in commercial areas.

> It has been a challenge for the company to keep the community and our workers motivated to participate in the program. We have to deal with diverse demands from the stakeholders and sometimes their other needs are more pressing. But we have nevertheless kept the program going.
>
> —K. K. Kaul, Executive Director, DSCL's Kota plant

Partnerships

The DSCL program has relied on partnerships from the outset. In designing the initial strategy, the official taking responsibility for the program consulted with area organizations that deal with HIV and AIDS, including industry associations and government entities. And those in the company who have implemented the program have often benefited from inputs from partners. These partners include:

- The Rajasthan State AIDS Control Society, the government organization responsible for the state AIDS program in Rajasthan.
- The Confederation of Indian Industry and its Social Development Council in the northern region. The council interacts with companies that are confederation members on issues of corporate social responsibility.
- The Energy and Resources Institute (TERI).

Funding

The program is funded entirely through internal resources of DSCL. Management allocates Rs 500,000 (around US$11,000) a year for the program through the annual budget. But if program needs exceed the allocated budget, management can approve additional support.

Outreach

Mass awareness programs at the workplace and in the surrounding community have covered about 75,000 people. These include contract workers, truck drivers and their assistants, and citizens of the city of Kota who visit the company during local festivals.

Lessons learned

The program has identified key factors in its success as well as key challenges and other lessons.

Key success factors

- *Management commitment.* The continued interest and involvement of senior management since the program's inception has been critical, providing the impetus and motivation for successful implementation. As noted, DSCL's HIV and AIDS intervention is financed by the company and thus has a greater likelihood of sustainability than if it depended on external sources of funding.
- *Enthusiasm and innovativeness of the responsible official.* The official responsible for the program was no expert on HIV and AIDS. But he devised unique strategies for the program by combining information from more knowledgeable sources with his own knowledge of the local area. This innovative spirit led to

> What gets monitored gets done.
>
> —Ajay S. Shriram, Chairman and Senior Managing Director, DSCL

interesting ways of spreading information, such as songs, poems, stories, and street plays (nukkad nataks) in the local dialect.

Key challenges

- *Stigma associated with HIV and AIDS in a conservative, semiurban area.* DSCL confronted ignorance, inhibitions, and misconceptions among the local population—and thus resistance to the HIV and AIDS program. The company's engagement with the local population to counter its fears and to persuade it that the program was in the interest of public health helped overcome the resistance.
- *Lack of infrastructure and potential partners.* Key challenges have been the inadequate government HIV and AIDS facilities in the area (the local government hospital has only a voluntary counseling and testing center, though staffed by a doctor) and the difficulty in finding local NGOs to act as effective project partners. The company overcame these obstacles by designing its own information, education, and communication material and relying on its own employees and occupational health team to spread awareness about HIV and AIDS.

Other lessons learned

- *Sensitivity to local culture and local sensibilities.* Using information, education, and communication material and dissemination mechanisms that suit local sensibilities helped the program gain acceptance among the local population.

- *Use of existing internal resources.* The program has benefited from DSCL employees' skills and capabilities in creating information, education, and communication material. Relying on employees rather than an external agency to create awareness about HIV and AIDS has also helped build a greater sense of ownership for the program within the company. This approach offers a good example of how to mainstream HIV and AIDS activities and might help in institutionalizing and sustaining the response over time.

Future plans

The company's future plans for its HIV and AIDS program, outlined in its initial strategy, cover several areas of effort.

The HIV prevention and detection plan calls for:

- Conducting awareness programs in the city of Kota for school-children, the police, and high-risk groups such as drug users and local jail inmates.
- Proactively distributing condoms.
- Conducting blood testing campaigns to detect HIV.
- Providing financial assistance to those suspected of being HIV-positive but who cannot afford the test to detect HIV.

The AIDS treatment plan includes:

- Providing antiretroviral drugs to those needing them.
- Providing financial assistance for nutritional enhancement for those undergoing treatment.

Finally, the rehabilitation plan covers several actions:

- Creating a nondiscriminatory environment in the workplace consistent with the company's HIV and AIDS policy.
- Transferring HIV-positive employees to positions involving less physical strain if that is important for their health.
- Partnering with other organizations to help AIDS patients earn income to support themselves and undergo treatment.

Case Study:
Hindustan Lever Limited

Overview

Hindustan Lever Limited (HLL), a leader in the fast-moving consumer goods business, is among the top five exporters in India.[15] HLL's distribution network, with more than 3,400 distributors and 16 million outlets, markets more than a thousand products manufactured in more than a hundred plants across India.

The company's HIV and AIDS program, initiated in 2002, focuses on protecting the health of its skilled young workforce. Its factories have HIV and AIDS awareness initiatives built into their health and safety training.

The program also extends beyond the workplace, spreading awareness about HIV and AIDS through two vehicles: Project Sanjivini, which provides medical care to the poor in remote villages of eastern India, and Project Shakti, which focuses on microcredit, training, and empowerment of women. Here HLL makes good use of its expertise in distribu-

---

15. The information in the HLL case study is based on HLL's response to a questionnaire sent to the company by email; a personal interview with the company's vice president for medical and occupational health at Mumbai; telephone conversations with the medical officers of the company's northern and southern regions; and HLL's 2005 annual report (HLL 2006). This information is current as of September 2006.

tion and management to work with rural entrepreneurs in spreading awareness.

Business background

HLL is a multinational company 51 percent owned by the Anglo-Dutch company Unilever. Its product portfolio features household and personal care products—including such leading household brands in India as Surf—as well as foods and beverages. The company distributes nearly a thousand products through its network of 4 warehouses, more than 40 agents, 7,500 wholesalers, and many large institutional customers. It also sources raw materials, intermediates, and packaging materials from more than 2,000 suppliers. Net sales in 2005 totaled US$2.2 billion.

Since the 1980s HLL has directed most of its investments to designated backward areas and zero-industry districts, helping to revive several sick industries and develop local entrepreneurship. The company also focuses on a range of community support activities, including water management, empowerment of women, and health and hygiene education.

Why do something about HIV and AIDS?

As a subsidiary of Unilever, HLL is committed to providing a safe and healthy working environment for all employees in accordance with both Unilever standards on occupational health and national and international public health regulations and requirements relating to HIV and AIDS. This commitment is reflected in the company's HIV and AIDS policy (box 3).

Box 3. The HIV and AIDS policy of HLL

In 2004 HLL formulated an HIV and AIDS policy that assures employees of a nondiscriminatory work environment and assistance in seeking appropriate treatment that is currently available. The overarching goal is to protect employees' health. The policy was drafted by HLL's Occupational Health Division under the Unilever HIV and AIDS guidelines and communicated to all employees as well as to supply chain partners, including suppliers and distributors.

Further impetus to strengthen HIV and AIDS awareness programs across all units came from the company's belief that the epidemic poses formidable challenges to development and social progress in India. The primary goals of HLL's program are to reduce absenteeism and health costs and increase productivity and life expectancy.

The program

HLL launched its HIV and AIDS initiative in 2002 in the units in its southern region. In 2004 it extended the initiative to its eastern and western regions, and in early 2005 to its northern region.

The basic approach in all HLL units includes reaching out to all employees and business partners through HIV and AIDS awareness programs and educating people living with HIV. But to ensure commitment from those implementing

> To succeed requires the highest standards of corporate behavior toward our employees, consumers, and the societies and the world in which we live. As a part of this corporate behavior HLL is strongly committed to ensure appropriate workplace prevention and control of HIV and AIDS, and we will share this expertise across the supply chain and communities among which we operate.
>
> —Douglas Baillie, Chief Executive Officer HLL, India and Group Vice President, South Asia, Unilever.

the program, the company allows each unit to improve or modify the program according to local needs.

In areas with a high national prevalence of HIV, such as those in the western and southern states, HLL units support comprehensive workplace programs that cover nondiscrimination, prevention education, access to counseling and testing, and care, support, and treatment. Units in areas less affected by the epidemic support community initiatives in HIV and AIDS education and awareness along with other health issues. Some HLL units have established voluntary blood testing for HIV antibodies. Many units distribute free condoms at strategic locations.

The HIV and AIDS program is spearheaded by HLL's occupational health team and Human Resources Department and implemented through its unit medical officers. All HLL units have occupational health centers with basic health facilities to treat patients with support from government-designated medical institutions.

HLL also makes continual efforts to build the skills of medical staff in different units. In collaboration with the Confederation of Indian Industry and the ILO, it has provided training for company physicians on issues relating to HIV and AIDS. In addition, the Confederation of Indian Industry and the National AIDS Control Organization conducted a "train the trainers" workshop for the medical staff. This workshop included discussions on the development and progression of HIV infection, disease monitoring including clinical criteria based on WHO specifications, and the latest diagnostic techniques. The company's medical staff has also received training in antiretroviral therapy and drug administration.

To ensure the success of the program at the unit level, each HLL unit integrates shop floor employees and managers into the core team, made up of the unit head, human resource personnel, shop floor manager, and a workforce representative. This core team is sensitized to HIV and AIDS issues at the beginning of the unit's program. The team participates in the quarterly review of the program undertaken in each unit, meeting with other partners if needed.

Awareness and prevention activities at the workplace

Southern and western regions

HLL's workplace program in the southern and western regions consists of group awareness programs, training of peer educators, and sensitization of general employees. Units conduct programs in both English and local languages in collaboration with district health authorities, local AIDS cells (government bodies responsible for HIV prevention and control activities), and voluntary organizations (picture 11). The units also conduct

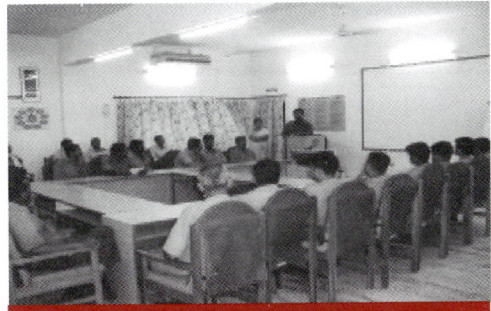

Picture 11. Session being conducted at the Mangalore unit by the doctor who is the officer in charge of the local voluntary counseling and testing center

awareness programs for truckers and contract workers through posters, audiovisual sessions, mass education activities, information booklets in regional languages, and interactions with neighboring industries.

Since HLL's southern region has had a few reported cases of HIV infection, the company introduced voluntary blood testing in 25 units in the region. Managers lead the way in the testing to set an example for others (pictures 12 and 13). While the company keeps an aggregate record of these blood tests at the unit level, it maintains a high level of confidentiality for individual employees and contract workers.

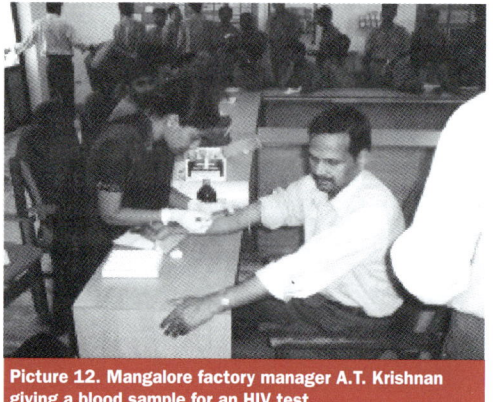

Picture 12. Mangalore factory manager A.T. Krishnan giving a blood sample for an HIV test

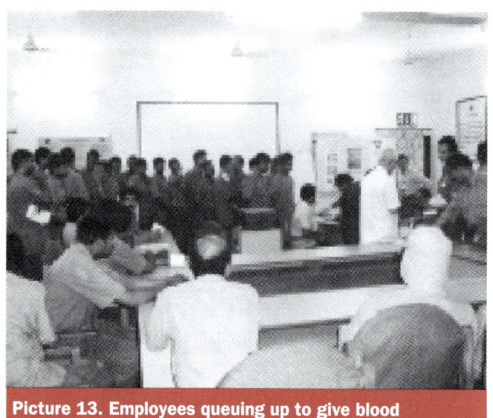

Picture 13. Employees queuing up to give blood samples for HIV testing at the Mangalore factory

The company allows paid leave for employees requiring medical attention for HIV or AIDS. More important, it also provides support and counseling to their family during the treatment period.

Northern region

HLL's northern region, whose eight units together are the largest supplier of HLL products across India, received support from the ILO for its HIV and AIDS initiative. The program informed top management about the HIV situation in India and educated employees about how to reduce risky behavior and contribute to a discrimination free work environment. In addition, an initial sensitization session with the ILO briefed all unit heads and human resource managers on how to implement an HIV and AIDS program.

The northern region also sought ILO's technical assistance to reach out to other companies within the group and to supply chain partners. HLL has signed a memorandum of understanding with the ILO on the plan for implementing the HIV and AIDS awareness program. And NGOs trained by the ILO are conducting a knowledge, attitude, beliefs, and practices (KABP) survey in all northern regional units under a time-bound action plan.

Interventions for the community

In the southern region HLL implements focused awareness programs and promotes and distributes condoms among high-risk groups in the community. At the Tea Estate Division in Valparai, Tamil Nadu, for example, the company initiated a voluntary screening program for HIV and conducts special HIV and AIDS awareness programs for high-risk groups. The program also includes screening for all pregnant women at the end of their second trimester and in routine surgical cases among company employees.

The eastern region, in Assam, reports having had no cases of HIV. But units in the region hold training classes on HIV and AIDS awareness and also provide general medical care. The HLL factory in Doom Dooma, Assam, has formed local partnerships to provide basic medical services in remote villages that lack access to modern health facilities. This is done through an HLL-funded medical project, Sanjivini, through which the company supplied two am-bulances. The project holds Sanjivini camps, where the vans visit remote villages and provide basic medical services (picture 14). This project aims to reach out to 70,000 people in remote villages. The project also conducts a range of health awareness programs in associa-tion with local district authori-

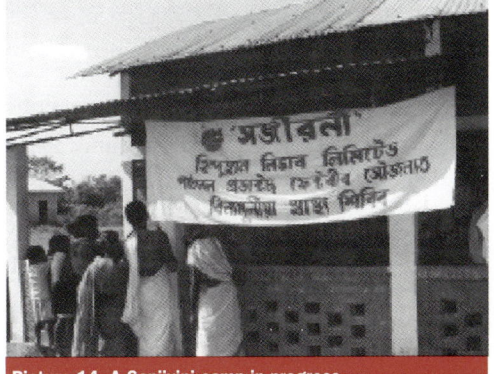

Picture 14. A Sanjivini camp in progress

Box 4. Reaching rural villages through Project Shakti

In 2001 HLL initiated Project Shakti in Nalgonda district, Andhra Pradesh, to provide microcredit and to train women to become direct-to-home distributors through self-help groups in rural areas. As an extension of this project, HLL set up Internet kiosks—commonly referred to as "iShakti"—in these rural areas to disseminate information in local languages, including material on health education.

Today Project Shakti has spread to 15 Indian states, reaching 85,000 villages in 385 districts through 20,000 female entrepreneurs, or "Shakti ammas." The distribution network formed by these female entrepreneurs could in the future distribute condoms in rural areas. HLL estimates that by 2010 the network will grow to around 100,000 trained women covering 50,000 villages.

---

ties. The company hopes to use Sanjivini to spread knowledge about HIV and AIDS to these remote communities.

Another HLL-funded initiative, Project Shakti, distributes health information in rural areas. And it holds promise for playing a far larger role in the future (box 4).

Partnerships

Each HLL unit relies on partnerships to implement the company's HIV and AIDS and health programs. Partners include:

- Medical college hospitals, for clinical expertise.
- The Confederation of Indian Industry, the ILO, and the National AIDS Control Organization, for training support.
- Community opinion leaders.

- Local NGOs.
- Public health officials.
- Neighboring industries.

These partnerships ensure local and government involvement. Moreover, by integrating HLL's HIV and AIDS initiative with local organizations and with the company's overall health program, they help the company gain credibility with its employee base and the general community.

Funding

Since occupational health is a priority for HLL, the corporate budget for HIV and AIDS initiatives is flexible. That allows units to function with some independence. It also makes it possible to give units support for unbudgeted expenses on short notice if needed.

> Given our large workforce, it does not make business sense for us to engage in a group medical policy or similar insurance or medical schemes. It is better to provide complete care and treatment for the needy may it be for HIV and AIDS or any other ailment.
>
> —Dr. T. Rajgopal, Vice President, Medical and Occupational Health, HLL

Lessons learned

The program has several observations about the key factors in its success and its key challenges.

Key success factors

- *Management-led initiative.* HLL's management-led initiative has been a critical factor in ensuring sustainability of the HIV and AIDS program to date.
- *Commitment at all levels.* Allowing each unit to develop initiatives and providing budgetary support as needed ensure commitment to the program at all levels.

Key challenges

- *Overcoming stigma.* Employees initially were reluctant to take condoms, though distributed at no cost, because of the stigma attached to the use of condoms. Repeated awareness programs helped to overcome this resistance. The company also faced initial difficulty in gaining acceptance of voluntary testing. Repeated sessions again helped, convincing stakeholders of the importance of testing. Unit heads, managers, and officers also helped by leading the way at the voluntary testing sessions.

Future plans

HLL wishes to further extend its HIV and AIDS program through its distribution network. It would also like to improve health care in rural areas through its strong network of female entrepreneurs, known as "Shakti ammas." Before the program is expanded, it will be important to evaluate its effectiveness.

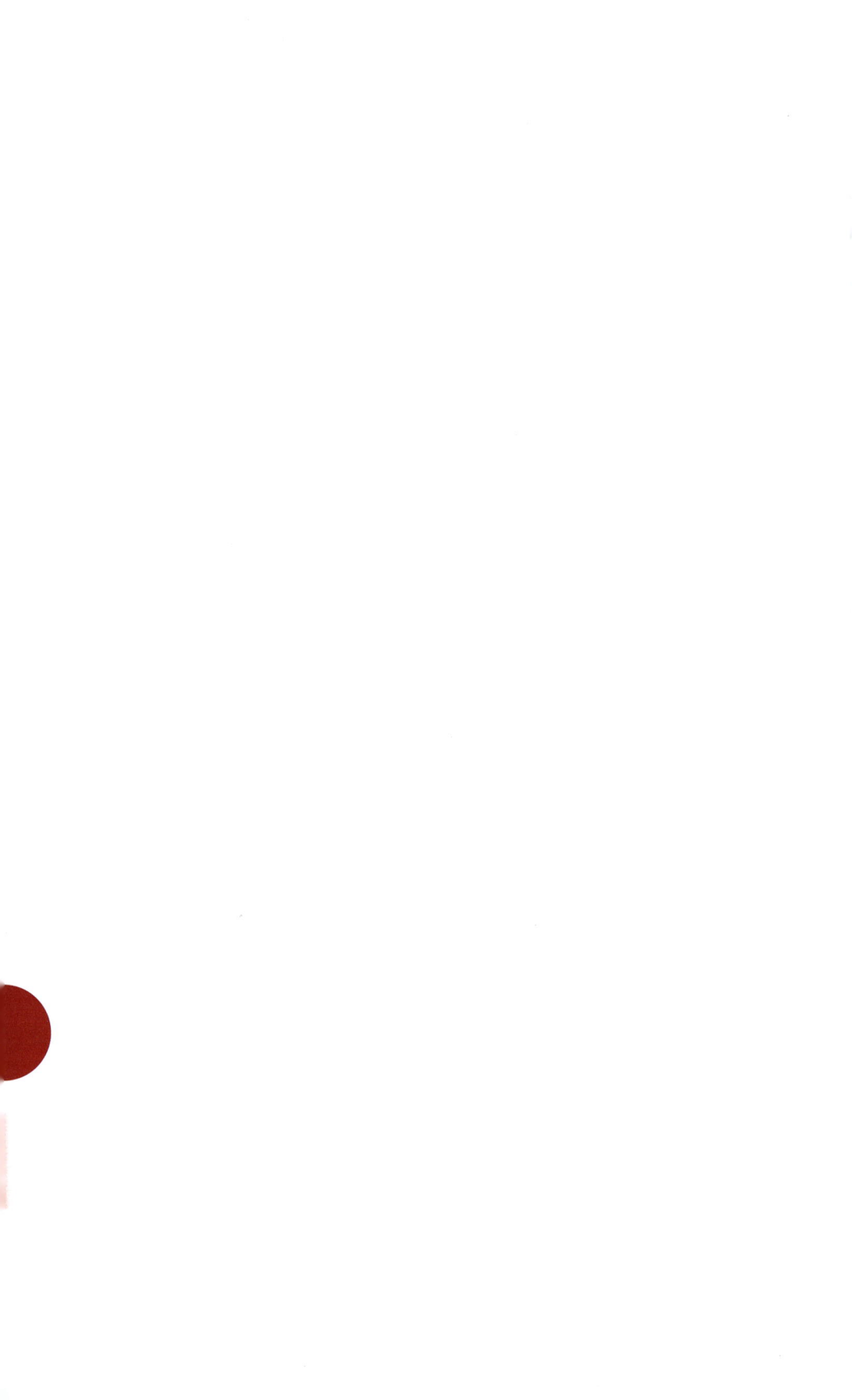

References

Chandrasekaran, Padma, Gina Dallabetta, Virginia Loo, Sujata Rao, Helene Gayle, and Ashok Alexander. 2006. "Containing HIV/AIDS in India: The Unfinished Agenda." *The Lancet Infectious Diseases* 6 (8): 508–21.

HLL (Hindustan Lever Limited). 2006. *Annual Report 2005*. Mumbai.

India, Ministry of Finance. 2006. "Foreign Exchange Reserves." In *Union Budget 2005–06*. New Delhi. http://indiabudget.nic.in/es2005-06/chapt2006/chap617.pdf.

JBIC (Japan Bank for International Cooperation). 2005. "Addressing Social Concerns Related to Project Undertakings." In *JBIC Environmental and Social Activities Report*. Tokyo.

LVS (Lok Vikas Sanstha). 2004. "STD Prevalence in Hazira." Surat, Gujarat.

Modicare Foundation. 2006. "HIV/AIDS Intervention with Migrant Workers: Project Undertaken by Delhi Metro Rail Corporation Ltd." Delhi.

Moses, Stephen, James F. Blanchard, Han Kang, Faran Emmanuel, Sushena Reza Paul, Marissa L. Becker, David Wilson, and Mariam Claeson. 2006. AIDS in South Asia: Understanding and Responding to a Heterogeneous Epidemic. Washington, D.C.: World Bank.

UNAIDS (Joint United Nations Programme on HIV/AIDS). 2006. *Report on the Global AIDS Epidemic 2006*. New York.

VHAI (Voluntary Health Association of India). 2003. "Study Awareness Campaign for Mitigation of HIV/AIDS Risks under Delhi Mass Rapid Transport System Project." Delhi.

World Bank. 2006. "The Business Case for AIDS." South Asia Multi Sector Briefs on HIV/AIDS. June. South Asia Region, Finance and Private Sector, Washington, D.C.

Company Web sites

- DCM Shriram Consolidated Limited: http://www.dscl.com/
- Delhi Metro Rail Corporation: http://www.delhimetrorail.com/index.htm
- Hindustan Lever Limited: http://www.hll.com/
- Reliance Industries Limited: http://www.ril.com/
- Transport Corporation of India: http://www.tcil.com/

Other Web sites

- Avahan: http://www.gatesfoundation.org/GlobalHealth/Pri_Diseases/HIVAIDS/HIVProgramsPartnerships/Avahan.htm
- IFC Against AIDS: http://www.ifc.org/ifcext/aids.nsf/content/home
- International Labour Organization: http://www.ilo.org/
- National AIDS Control Organization: http://www.nacoonline.org/
- SAR AIDS: http://www.worldbank.org/saraids
- UNAIDS India: http://www.unaids.org.in
- World Bank Institute: http://www.worldbank.org/wbi

Eco-Audit

Environmental Benefits Statement

The World Bank is committed to preserving Endangered Forests and natural resources. The Office of the Publisher has chosen to print *Corporate Responses to HIV/AIDS* on 25 percent postconsumer recycled paper, FSC certified. The World Bank has formally agreed to follow the recommended standards for paper usage set by Green Press Initiative—a nonprofit program supporting publishers in using fiber that is not sourced from Endangered Forests. For more information, visit www.greenpressinitiative.org.

In 2004, the printing of these books on recycled paper saved the following:

Trees*	Solid Waste	Water	Net Greenhouse Gases	Electricity
3	116	1,006	307	2
'40' in height and 6-8" in diameter	Pounds	Gallons	Pounds	Million BTUs

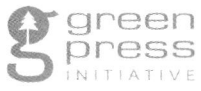